Praise for
The Insider's Guide to
Mental Health Resources Online

"From beginners to people who are fairly computer literate, but not fluent, to the really fluent computer user, this is a very useful guide that will probably save hours of endless search and information overload on the Internet."
—*The Scientific and Medical Network*

"A renowned psychologist and Internet expert shares his secrets for successfully searching the Internet to find information useful for professional mental health providers. An approachable style, insightful annotations, and four-star rating system make this the most important Internet guide for users seeking mental health information online....Grohol's presentation of Internet ethical considerations for psychologists is particularly useful. Recommended."   —*Choice*

"A wonderful book to peruse and keep on one's desk for ideas about 'where to look next.'...This book is great because of its wealth of information and pointers to where one can find additional information. I can only imagine how hard it is to write about a subject that is best taught and explained by one's personal experience. This book makes a good starting point for a mental health professional's online experience."
—*Metapsychology Online Book Reviews*

"This book offers thousands of tips for using the Internet to locate information and resources on mental health issues." —*Journal of the History of the Behavioral Sciences*

"Although Grohol has geared his book for the mental health practitioner, it is extremely useful for undergraduate or graduate students, researchers, or librarians in any health-related field. What makes it different from so many other Internet search guides is its extensive coverage of search engines plus an entire chapter on how to put together a successful search strategy....Even experienced searchers will find tips on how to use search engines effectively and will appreciate the author's candid opinions on which sites are a waste of time."   —*American Reference Books Annual*

The Insider's Guide to Mental Health Resources Online

THE CLINICIAN'S TOOLBOX™

A Guilford Series

EDWARD L. ZUCKERMAN, Series Editor

The Insider's Guide to Mental Health Resources Online, Revised Edition

JOHN M. GROHOL

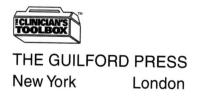

THE GUILFORD PRESS
New York   London

© 2004 The Guilford Press
A Division of Guilford Publications, Inc.
72 Spring Street, New York, NY 10012
www.guilford.com

Printed in the United States of America

This book is printed on acid-free paper.

Last digit is print number: 9 8 7 6 5 4 3 2 1

ISBN 1-57230-988-1

In memory of Rob & Anne

About the Author

John M. Grohol, PsyD, is a Boston-area author, online expert, and researcher. He built drkoop.com's Mental Health Center and was the cofounder and director for nearly 4 years of Mental Help Net, at one time one of the top 10 most-trafficked mental health Web sites. As one of the youngest chief operating officers in the behavioral health care industry, he oversaw the continuing development of HelpHorizons.com, an e-therapy services provider. He is currently a senior Web architect and founder of an Internet consulting and Web services company, Liviant LLC.

Trained and educated as a clinical psychologist at Nova Southeastern University, he has been a patient advocate, mental health educator, and online services innovator. While he has been involved in online services as early as 1981, he began on the Internet in 1991 as a regular contributor to the Internet's discussion forums, Usenet newsgroups. He has founded and moderated a number of newsgroups since then, including sci.psychology.research and sci.psychology.announce.

As one of the pioneering leaders in psychology online, Dr. Grohol was the editor-in-chief and founder of *Perspectives: A Mental Health Magazine,* an associate editor of *Behavior OnLine* and the bimonthly newsletter *PsychNews International,* and an associate editor for the print journal *Journal of Technology in Human Services.* He was a visiting instructor for 3 years with the Department of Epidemiology and Social Medicine, Albert Einstein College of Medicine, and is on the faculty at the Cape Cod Institute. He has chaired and presented at nearly three dozen symposia about online mental health and psychology at American Psychological Association conventions, for the Cape Cod Institute, and for Behavioral Informatics Tomorrow (where he also was an advisory board member).

Dr. Grohol sits on the editorial boards for the *Journal of Online Behavior* and *CyberPsychology & Behavior*. He is a founding member and the first president of the International Society for Mental Health Online (ISMHO) and sits on the advisory board of the Institute of Cybermedicine, affiliated with the Department of Psychiatry at Harvard Medical School. Dr. Grohol has had media appearances on *Good Morning America*, CNN & Time, *The Crier Report*, and local broadcasts. He maintains his own Web site at PsychCentral.com and has hosted a free weekly mental health chat online since 1995.

Acknowledgments

A book of this undertaking could not have been accomplished without the help of many people, to whom I owe a great deal. Thanks to The Guilford Press, Ed Zuckerman, and Barbara Watkins for recognizing the potential of this book and skillfully guiding it through the publishing process. Thanks to Tom Ferguson and Ed Madara for providing me with the model, motivation, and words of encouragement to take on this project. I am grateful to CMHC Systems, John Paton, and David Chrestay for providing me with the time and resources necessary to disseminate my knowledge in writing and expand my work online. Thanks to my parents, Lillian and Paul, for their encouragement, support, and love, imbuing within me the ability to achieve my simple goal in life: helping others. I would also like to thank my dearest Nancy, for she is a familiar soul who has been my inspiration and muse. I have never known such joy and peace than with her by my side.

stay on top of what's on the net...on the net

Visit the "Insider's Guide" online update page to stay current on additions and changes to the resources in this edition.

www.insidemh.com

Foreword

One cannot escape hearing about the Internet and today it is relatively easy to get "on the net." But what will mental health professionals find there that enables them to do their work better? When I first got online, I spent several dozen hours "surfing the net." It was exciting and entertaining but did not make me a better psychologist. Then I found Dr. Grohol's site, and he pointed me to the treasures. (You can find his site now at `http://grohol.com`.)

If anyone is an expert on the online world, surely it is Dr. Grohol. I e-mailed my appreciation for his helpful advice and out of that initial contact has developed this superb guide to the net's riches.

There are hundreds of books on the Internet and several that deal in some way with the mental health area. But, as you would expect from an Internet expert who is also a psychologist, this book is a treasure house of professional riches. He is not content simply to offer us lists of the many fine materials on the net. He goes on to share with us how he, as a clinician, really uses the net. He shows us all the searching techniques he uses to find resources to enrich his professional activities. With his expert guidance, you will learn to use the many "search engines" effectively, to join mailing lists of colleagues who share your specific interests, to find online jounals with the most up-to-date information, and where to post your questions on electronic "bulletin boards" to tap into the collective wisdom of the mental health community.

He shows us how to find answers to the kinds of everyday clinical and research questions we have. Best of all, as we accompany him on his search and learn the actual methods he uses, he tells us which are the sites most worth our professional time.

This book is indeed the "Insider's Guide" we need to the world of the net. It gently and clearly guides our exploring, making the trip both productive and pleasant. It takes us to destinations local and all over the globe. It introduces us to colleagues who share our interests and invites productive dialogues. Like the best of guidebooks, it excites with its promises, touches us with it personal relevance, and educates us as travellers.

EDWARD L. ZUCKERMAN, PhD

Contents

The Insider's Guide to
Mental Health Resources Online

Basic Map and Tools for Finding Mental Health Information Online

1

Why and How to Look Online

As a professional, you no doubt find the demands on your time are increasing. Managed care is loudly knocking on clinicians' doors. Universities are demanding more of faculty but offering less. Grant funding through federal government agencies is drying up. You have probably never worked harder and longer for less money. So it's no surprise that professionals are looking to maximize the value of the limited time they can spend online. There's no time to become familiar with this new landscape and use it effectively in your day-to-day job. Furthermore, you've probably heard many different things about getting online, including: "I hear of people getting online and simply getting lost!"; "Why should I waste my time?"; "I've heard it can be frustrating and expensive."

It *is* easy to get lost online if you don't know where to look for information. In this book, I show you where to go to find what you need professionally.

It takes an immense amount of time to discover what's available and where to find it online. I have already done that—with you, the professional, in mind. Out of the myriad resources available online, how do you know what is good and worth your professional time? In this book, I give you my assessments of quality and rate each online resource. With these tools in hand, you can *choose* your best bet, rather than having to stumble upon it.

WHAT'S AVAILABLE ONLINE FOR YOU?

How can online resources help you, the mental health professional? Communication and convenience are two significant assets. Communication with other professionals—not just across the nation, but across the world—is quick, easy, and cheap online. E-mail (electronic mail) allows this, providing greater collaborative possibilities for research and clinical case consultation. For example, clinicians or researchers working alone or in remote or rural areas can now present difficult or challenging cases to their international colleagues to get useful feedback on treatment approaches. Questions about new medications coming on the market can be answered by experts within the psychopharmacology field who maintain Internet mailing lists. E-mail and mailing lists are described in greater depth later in this chapter.

While communication is the key to many professionals' choosing to get online, increased convenience in accessing information resources is often the reason professionals stay. Most academics and clinicians cannot access databases such as MEDLINE or PsycINFO without making a trip to the university library. But such databases are easily accessible online and, in some cases, free. Not everyone has a copy of the *Physicians' Desk Reference* (PDR) ready to hand. Resources similar to the PDR are available online. In-depth clinical and research articles and references, which summarize the major treatment approaches and latest research developments for any given disorder, can be browsed online. The *Diagnostic and Statistical Manual of Mental Disorders* (DSM) diagnostic codes and *International Classification of Diseases* (ICD) definitions of mental disorders are available at your fingertips online. Going online gives you access to all kinds of information easily and conveniently. How many libraries are open 24 hours a day, 365 days a year?

As a clinician online, you will be able to consult on difficult cases; learn about new theories, therapies, methods, and assessment measures; and talk to colleagues with similar therapeutic interests around the world (see Chapters 4, 6, and 7). As a researcher, you can collaborate with other researchers on the same study much easier than in the past, with the use of e-mail and the World Wide Web. New information can often be obtained more easily online, through news resources, current tables of contents for relevant journals, and databases (see Chapters 3, 7, and 9). The Web offers connections to such information, research and medical databases, and many similar resources. And because the entire Web is searchable, finding all of this information is much easier than you might think. Journal articles will sometimes be available by subscription, as well as news updates through a professional organization's Web site. Continuing education calendars are available online, and some online continuing education courses allow you to take courses at your leisure, and at greatly reduced costs (Chapter 5). You can find professional employment opportunities online (Chapter 4), discover the wealth of psychological software available (Chapter 10), and obtain patient education resources and materials (Chapters 12, 13, and 14).

WHAT'S NOT AVAILABLE ONLINE (YET)

When I first wrote this book in 1996, a great deal of information was not yet available online. Much has changed since then, with some journal publishers embracing the Internet and allowing subscribers online access to articles. Although it is not clear that the vast majority of older journal articles will ever make it online, those published in the past few years and those published currently often have electronic versions available. Some journals provide online access to their articles as a part of their base subscription fee, and others charge extra for such access. Initiatives such as the National Institutes of Health's PubMed Central provides an online, free public archive of life science journal articles, some dating back to 1994 (see `http://www.pubmedcentral.nih.gov/`). Notably absent from this archive, however, are psychology, social work, and psychiatry journals. However, such archives have the potential to provide a rich array of readily available, free scientific articles to consume.

One of the world's largest medical databases is freely available online (MEDLINE). What many mental health professionals don't realize is that it includes most of the larger and better-known social science and psychological journal abstracts. So although proprietary, commercial databases such as the American Psychological Association's PsycINFO are also available online for the right cost (if you cannot obtain access through a local university's library), many times the free MEDLINE database will suffice for quick literature searches.

ABOUT THIS BOOK

Throughout this book I highlight not only the key resources but also some of the lesser-known corners of the online world, to give you the insider's perspective to what is available online. The book is arranged into three major parts. This first part orients you to the online world and shows you how to make it work for you. It gives advice on formulating questions that get useful results, and where best to look for the answers. I also offer a step-by-step search strategy. The second part addresses the specific topics professionals are likely to want more information about. These topics range from how to find a job to where to look for cognitive therapy resources. If what you are looking for is not specifically covered in Part II, the tools and resources described in Part I and throughout the book should enable you to find it. The third part helps clinicians help their clients find online resources for patient education and self-help.

Appendix A offers a glossary of terms used throughout this book. There are many books about the Internet that devote entire chapters to the basics of getting online and the differences between online commercial service providers. I believe these are useful things to know, but I do not spend a lot of time covering them. For more information, I refer the reader to the publications in Appendix B. See Appendix C for a brief guide to getting online. Appendix D discusses how to create a simple World Wide Web page of your own.

If you're new to the whole online world, I suggest you read Appendix C first, get online successfully, and then continue with the rest of this book. Specific information about the minimal computer requirements for making the most out of online resources is discussed in the accompanying box as well as in Appendix C. The key to accessing online resources is not the computer you use, but the speed of your connection to the online world. While I try to be as non–computer specific and unbiased as possible throughout the book, I conduct all of my work online with an IBM-PC compatible computer. Where appropriate, I make reference to software that is computer spe-

MINIMAL COMPUTER REQUIREMENTS FOR MAKING THE MOST OF YOUR ONLINE EXPERIENCE

While you can use almost any computer to access many online resources, your online experience will be best if your computer setup meets the following minimal technical requirements. See Appendix C for a more thorough description and discussion of these requirements.

Your Computer:

- An IBM-PC compatible computer with an Intel or Pentium-class processor running at 133 MHz minimum or

- a Macintosh II, Quadra, Performa, PowerPC of any kind, G3, G4, or iMac.

- Memory: 32 MB of RAM for Windows 95/98/ME
  64 MB of RAM for Windows NT/2000/XP
  or Macintosh System 8, 9, or X

- Hard disk space: 100 MB available (free)

Your Modem:

- An internal or external modem running at 33.6 Kbps minimum, although 56 Kbps is strongly recommended; or a cable, satellite, or DSL modem.

Online Access:

- An Internet service provider (local or national) or online commercial service provider (such as America OnLine or CompuServe)

cific. One of the nicest advantages to the online world, though, is that *it really doesn't matter* what kind of computer or operating system you use to access it. The online resources will generally work and look the same. The next part of this chapter gives a basic orientation to the important areas in the online world: e-mail, newsgroups, the World Wide Web, and search engines. If you already know about each of these, you might want to skip ahead. But don't skip the "Security Online" section that ends this chapter.

While I have gone to great pains to ensure the timeliness and accuracy of all the resources listed throughout the book, electronic addresses do change from time to time. Please check out the book's Web site (`http://www.insidemh.com/`) for updates.

THE MAJOR RESOURCES IN THE ONLINE WORLD

The online world is made up of millions of computers in thousands of locations throughout the world. It consists not only of the popular World Wide Web, but of many other older and less glamorous resources, including simple e-mail, newsgroups, mailing lists, interactive real-time chat rooms, and much more. I highlight the resources most actively used by professionals online today, outlining them briefly below.

About E-Mail

The easiest and most widely-used aspect of being online is called "electronic mail," or "e-mail" for short. As the name implies, this is an electronic version of regular mail, though it is not as secure (see cautions below). E-mail comes to your own electronic mail box, usually supplied as a service of your online access provider. At the cost of a local phone call, it allows a rapid, convenient method of corresponding and communicating with others around the world.

E-mail is also a gateway to online discussion areas called "mailing lists." Mailing lists (also known as "listservs" for the software that runs them) are where e-mail messages on specific areas of interest are publicly distributed. Many professionals-only mailing lists exist online to discuss specific mental health and behavioral health care topics. Each mailing list focuses on a specific topic. These can range from addictions and affective disorders to traumatic stress, psychotherapy treatment and research, and more. See Chapter 6 for a more detailed discussion of specific professional mailing lists together with a step-by-step guide on how to join—or "subscribe"—to them.

Once subscribed, you automatically receive a copy in your e-mail box of any message other members send to the list. You may simply read the messages then delete them, or you and other subscribers may choose to respond. These responses are also sent to every subscriber. In this manner, an interactive discussion can take place among the participants of the mailing list.

Cautions

E-mail is not as secure a method of correspondence as regular mail. The latter carries with it criminal charges for tampering. While online etiquette ("netiquette") dictates that e-mail is not to be shared publicly unless both parties first agree, the reality is that e-mail may be made public with little recourse if one party decides to do so. E-mail is adequate for most communications with your colleagues, but I'd never send credit card or other confidential information through it, unless encryption, a way of sending secure information online, is used.

Spam

Unsolicited commercial e-mail, also known as "spam," is a widespread problem for nearly all Internet users today. Until national governments make sending such unwanted commercial advertisements illegal, they will continue unabated. Why? Because it costs the advertising companies virtually nothing to send a spam e-mail message to you. Even if 99.999% of people who receive such an email simply dispose of it or never read it, the tiny percentage of people who act on the spam or buy the advertising company's product make it worthwhile for the company to continue this notorious marketing method. As long as no legitimate companies use spam, as is now the case, it is more likely to be outlawed. Keep in mind, however, that even after spam is made illegal, it will likely continue because the cost of enforcement will initially be tremendous.

While we are waiting for our governments to react against spammers (companies who send such unsolicited e-mail), it is easy to take action of your own. Nearly every type of modern e-mail software available for computers today has filtering capability. Some e-mail programs, such as the one built into the open-source, free Web browser called Mozilla (which you can download at `http://www.mozilla.org/`) have spam filters built in.

Not all e-mail programs have built-in spam filters, however, such as one of the most popular e-mail programs–Microsoft Outlook. A way of extending your e-mail software's filtering capabilities to greatly reduce spam is through a technology called "plug-ins." Plug-ins are simply specific filtering rules that can detect spam either before or after you download it to your computer, and which delete all e-mail that is likely spam. Some of these plug-ins have a 98% to 99.5% success rate in detecting spam from regular e-mail you receive. A useful, free plug-in for Outlook is called SpamBayes (`http://spambayes.sourceforge.net/`). I use an e-mail program called Eudora, and a quality spam plug-in for it is Spamnix (`http://www.spamnix.com/`). Spamnix offers a free download and 30-day trial period, but costs $29.95 to continue using it.

Check your e-mail program's documentation, as it may already have spam filtering available. If not, typing a query into a search engine such as Google (`http://www.google.com/`) will quickly locate many alternative spam filtering programs. For instance, if you were looking for spam filters available for Microsoft Outlook Express, you might try typing:

```
"spam filter" "outlook express" download
```

You will get dozens of results of programs that you can download to try for yourself.

Be certain to read the instructions for your spam filter, because such filters vary greatly in how they work. Some require training in order to be most effective, whereas others are more transparent in their operation. By installing a spam filter on your computer, you will quickly discover the joys of reading an Inbox devoid of most of the annoying spam that has become so commonplace online today.

About Newsgroups

"Newsgroups" (also known as "Usenet" or "Usenet newsgroups," their proper name) are also public discussion forums on the Internet. Unlike mailing lists, you access them through special software called a "news reader." News reading software is built into your Web browser or your e-mail software (such as Outlook). Newsgroups' advantages over mailing lists is that the format naturally supports "threading." A threaded discussion is one where you can read all of the messages on a particular topic more easily because they follow one another in order under that topic's title. Mailing lists, on the other hand, rely on your e-mail software to support threading. Users can also choose to delete entire threads in which they have no interest.

Newsgroups' advantage is disappearing because of new advances in e-mail software. As well, newsgroups also have their pitfalls. They are more public and easily accessible to everyone, and so everyone uses them. That makes some of them very busy. In addition to the high volume of messages, most newsgroups do not have any supervision or ownership (unlike mailing lists). This lack of supervision can result in a great deal of irrelevant and off-topic discussions. "Moderated" newsgroups help offset this problem, because messages must first be reviewed for appropriateness to the newsgroup's specific topic area before being published.

Newsgroups are categorized hierarchically by broad topic areas (e.g., recreational, science, computers, miscellaneous), which are then broken down into more specific subjects (e.g., psychology, medicine, physics), which are further broken down into still more discrete categories. For example, one newsgroup is named

```
sci.psychology.research
```

Each period, or "dot," denotes hierarchical level. "Sci" tells us this newsgroup is in the "science" hierarchy, under the subcategory of "psychology." This specific newsgroup, then, appears to be related to research topics in psychology. Newsgroups are generally much broader in scope and content than mailing lists are. They are also readily accessible through the Web at Google Groups (`http://groups.google.com`).

About the World Wide Web

E-mail and newsgroups are good for exchanging words but not images. The Web does both. The World Wide Web (also known simply as "the Web") is easily the most popular yet least interactive of online resources. Its popularity springs from the ease with which people can access it and the information found there. The Web was the first freely available Internet resource that allowed for the reproduction of graphics. Before the Web, the display of graphics online was generally a rare and tedious process. Graphics can still take a long time to be displayed because of their size and your connection speed to the online world. In the chapters that follow, I try to note when graphics may present a problem. The Web made it easy for anyone not only to access text and graphics, but also to create their own Web presence for others to access. (I will discuss how to create *your* own Web presence in Appendix D.)

The Web is made up of places called "Web sites" or "home pages." Some people use these terms interchangably, though I prefer to use the term "home page" to refer specifically to the first screen that is displayed when you access a Web site. A Web site is a person's or organization's entire Web offering, which may be made up of no more than one screen (called a "page" in Web lingo) of text information. More elaborate and larger Web sites might contain hundreds or thousands of individual Web pages, each with dozens of graphics. The most successful Web sites online today find a balance between judicious use of graphics and a great deal of original and useful content.

Web Site and E-Mail Addresses

Web sites have addresses, just like homes and businesses do in the real world. Web site addresses take the form of a URL (uniform resource locator) that contains several parts: (1) the name of the network protocol required to access the resource, (2) a domain name that identifies a specific, remote computer on the Internet, and (3) a file or directory location on that computer. This is best explained by looking at a sample Web address, such as:

```
http://www.nmha.org/index.cfm
```

The network protocol (in Web addresses, this is the `http://` component) tells your Web browser how to communicate with the remote computer. For the World Wide Web, this communication is through the HyperText Transfer Protocol (HTTP). The domain name (in Web addresses, this is the `www.nmha.org` component) tells the Internet's addressing system to look for this specific remote server on the Internet and connect to it, rather like looking up a phone number in the telephone book. The last component, `index.cfm`, is a specific file that you are requesting to retrieve from the remote computer. Once found on the remote computer, the file is downloaded and displayed within your Web browser.

All Web addresses are case sensitive, meaning that you must type in the address in upper- and lowercase letters exactly as shown. So while `http://www.nih.gov/news/` takes you to the National Institutes of Health's News and Events page, `http://www.nih.gov/NEWS/` will give you an error message. Most *e-mail addresses,* however, are not case sensitive; that is, it does not matter whether you type the address in upper- or lowercase letters. For example, `john@grohol.com` and `JOHN@GROHOL.COM` would both be properly delivered. Newsgroup addresses are also not case sensitive.

Many people receive Web addresses in an e-mail. Most e-mail programs allow you to click directly on the Web address while reading the e-mail message, which will bring up that Web site in your Web browser. You can also copy-and-paste the address into your Web browser's "Address" box. In either case, however, beware if there's a period found at the end of an address (because the address appeared at the end of a sentence, for example). You must manually remove that period in the Web address box in your Web browser before going to the site, or your Web browser may report an error.

Web Browsers

Your computer accesses the Web through a piece of software called a "Web browser." Web addresses (URLs) are typed into your Web browser and it, in turn, will find and display Web sites, including graphics and text. Browsers are available for any computer and operating system: One of the two most popular is published by Netscape, a division of America Online and is called "Netscape." Microsoft Corporation's "Internet Explorer" is the other most popular. Both are available online and at your local computer store. The Microsoft browser is included with their operating system, Windows , so you may already have it. Web browsers allow you to mark Web sites you like. Called "bookmarks" or "favorites," this feature allows you to save and subsequently easily access the address of a site. Some Web browsing software also have news readers and e-mail software built into them to enhance usability.

Once you are at any Web site, you navigate it by clicking on highlighted text or graphics called "links." When links are text, the word or phrase is often underlined or in a color different from the rest of the text on the screen. Whether text or graphics, you can recognize a link because your cursor will change into something other than an arrow (for instance, to a hand) when passed over it. For example, if you're reading about depression on a Web site, the terms "serotonin," "bipolar," and "suicide" may be highlighted as links. Clicking on any one link takes you to a new page—or even a new site—with more information on that topic. In this manner you can spend hours clicking on links, going from Web site to Web site, in search of additional information on a topic. This is what is meant by "surfing" the Web. The person responsible for maintaining a Web site is called a "Webmaster."

Web sites come in two major flavors—"framed" and "normal" (or unframed). A framed Web site is one in which your Web browser's screen is divided up into smaller screens (called "frames"), each of which contains different information. Some Web site designers do this to place a menu selection at the bottom or on the side of your Web browser's screen to help you navigate through the Web site more easily. Most Web browsers today can display frames. The drawback is that you generally need a larger screen to make the most use of them. On a too-small computer screen, you will be unable to see some of the information contained in one or more of the frames. Most Web sites in this book are of the normal, or unframed variety. When a framed version is offered or available, I will usually note that in the site's review. Even when a framed version of the Web site is offered, you can typically choose whether you want a framed or unframed version. The choice you make will probably depend on the opinion you form after trying out this feature on a few sites.

About Search Engines

One of the keys to making the Internet work *for* you is knowing how to use a search engine or guide. The online world is large and growing at an extraordinary rate. The amount of information to be searched, therefore, is also immense. While it is useful to know specific URLs and go directly to specific Web sites (or use your bookmarks), what else are you missing? Using a search engine, you can obtain a listing of possibly relevant sites and go directly to the site from the list. There are many different kinds of search engines, some better than others.

To use a search engine, type in a few words or topics you're interested in. Click on the "Search" button and the search engine will return some results. Results typically include the Web page's name or title, a summary or short description of the Web page, and a link directly to that page. You need only click on a result to go to that Web page.

The closest matches—that is, the most relevant documents found—will be listed first. The list is typically organized by declining relevancy—at least ideally. But different search engines have different algorithms for determining relevancy. The relevancy of the results to your initial query may vary greatly. For example, a story about a young woman who happened to read Freud's *Interpretation of Dreams*, may be indexed under "Freud." The hapless researcher types in "Freud" looking for biographical information, and the search engine returns this story about the young woman's reading material. If our researcher checks it out, she will have wasted time following an irrelevant path. Searching for information can often be a frustrating back-and-forth trudge from the search engine's list of results to the results themselves, most of which can turn out to be largely irrelevant to your intended purpose. But don't give up searching online. There are many useful and easy strategies to greatly enhance your search skills. See Chapter 2 for the different kinds of search engines available.

The Host of Other Internet Resources

There are many other resources I may mention throughout this book and you may hear about in your online travels. Some of these are covered in the glossary, found in Appendix A. The online world is so vast and expansive, it would be impossible for me to cover all the online resources that may have some relevance to professionals. For example, there are interactive, live chat rooms online in which people congregate 24 hours a day, 365 days a year. Most of these are for nonprofessionals, but there are a handful of areas like this where professionals occasionally meet. I expect that as more professionals discover the benefits of getting online, such live, interactive areas for professionals will increase in number.

FORMULATING QUESTIONS THAT GET RESULTS

Anyone who has done any type of research knows that formulating the right question is essential to getting useful answers. If the question is too vague or general, you may get little useful information. If the question is too narrowly defined, it may be impossible to generalize from your research findings. The same is true of searching for information online. If your search query is too broad, you will receive thousands of generally irrelevant results; if too narrow, you may not find anything at all. Either way, you'll probably become frustrated and give up. This section covers the tricks of the trade for searching for useful and relevant information online.

Most searching online is done *through* as well as *on* the World Wide Web. The results will be limited to information that has been published on the Web. (Some search engines can also search newsgroups—see Chapter 2.) There is a lag between the time a site is published on the Web and the time it is indexed. The Web has a tremendous size and growth rate—the indexing software simply cannot keep up. For example, if I publish a copy of my research on eating disorders on my Web site tomorrow, it may not be indexed by the Web indexing software for weeks or even months. While there are ways for authors and developers of Web sites to decrease this time lag, most do not actively do so. This means that while searching the Web is a potentially powerful tool, it should be just one of many such tools you use while online. I have sometimes discovered information in other online recesses, such as mailing lists, that don't exist on the Web (and therefore can't be found by a Web search engine).

Search Tools and Tips

Forming a Search Concept and Using Synonyms

Start a search by choosing a thorough and well-defined search concept. This concept should not only include your initial idea and its initial terms, but also include all terms related to that idea. Suppose we want to search for "teenage depression." That's our concept. If we just typed those two words into most search engines, we would be assaulted with thousands of relevant but also irrelevant results. For example, some search engines will automatically assume you're searching for the individual terms teenage *or* depression, but others will use teenage *and* depression. To get the most relevant results, you'll want to type in and between those two keywords.

Next we want to think of popular synonyms for these words, to ensure we gather *all* possibly relevant data. We will want the search engine to look for all these synonyms as well. For the search term "teenage," we may also want to include:

teenager
teenagers
adolescent
adolescents
youth

For "depression," we may also want to include:

suicide
depressed
loneliness
dysthymia
mood

We will want to search for each of the individual synonyms for teenage and depression. Therefore, you will want to type in o r between the synonyms for each word. The term and goes between the two sets of synonyms. Our search query is now expanded from "teenage and depression" to "(teenage or teenager or teenagers or adolescent or adolescents or youth) and (depression or suicide or depressed or loneliness or dysthymia or mood)." By using synonyms in this way, you can probably expand any search that is retrieving too few records (or too few *relevant* records). Notice the quotation marks and parentheses. They matter. The next section explains why.

By including all of the above choices, we can ensure that the search is the most thorough possible. This is no different from how most of us were taught to think about our queries before conducting a thorough literature search. For some reason, when professionals get online, they often forget these important lessons.

Tools for Precision Searching: Booleans, Phrases, and Other Operators

Ideally, we would like to search with greater precision and have fewer, but more relevant records returned. Search engines have been developed and equipped with tools to help increase the precision of a search. Some search engines' tools, however, are more powerful than others. It is these tools, *not the size of a search engine's database,* that make one search engine better than another. After all, what's the point of searching the largest library in the world if it has a poorly indexed card catalog? Unfortunately for you, each search engine has slightly different ways of implementing these tools, also known as "operators" in computer lingo.

Booleans   Most search engines allow you to insert the words "and," "or," and "not" to connect words or logical groupings of words. This is called "Boolean" searching and is the most basic search method. We've already used "and" and "or" in this way in our search for teenage depression. All search engines available today offer some means like this of limiting and broadening your searches. For instance, `mice` `and` `men` will retrieve items containing both terms, limiting the search, while `mice` `or` `men` will retrieve all items that have either term, broadening the search. `England` `not` `New` will provide you with items about England, but not about New England, thereby narrowing a search.

Phrases   A second method for helping you limit your search is through the use of "phrases." Search engines will recognize that words go together if you bracket them, for example, with quotation marks. The search engine will retrieve items that only match the specific phrase within the quotes. Typing quotes around `"teenage depression"` should be quite useful in retrieving results that discuss teenage depression. It should limit retrieval of documents that may use the words separately throughout that document, which can happen when using the Boolean operator `and`. The two main ways to indicate a phrase in a search engine is through the use of quotation marks or parentheses. Some search engines use one method and not the other, while some let you use both at the same time. Each search engine's help section offers additional information about which operators and punctuation they recognize (see Table 1.1). In our last search query for teenage depression, we created phrases with both quotation marks and parentheses. The quotations bracket the total concept with all the synonyms, while the parentheses contain the two sets of synonyms (much like a complex math equation!).

Other Operators   Additional tools (or "operators") are helpful in limiting or broadening our search. Like the Boolean terms, a word suggesting

TABLE 1.1   Quick Reference of Search Operators and Examples

Operator	Description	Example
and	Used between two or more search terms or expressions, **all** of which must appear in each result	`teenage and depression` will return only results with both the word "teenage" and the word "depression" in them
or	Used between two or more search terms or expressions, **any** of which may appear in each result	`teenage or depression` will return results with either of these two words in them
not	Used between two or more search terms or expressions; acts to exclude the search term or expression following it	`depression not teenage` will exclude any depression-related results that have the word "teenage" in them
"..."	Used around a group of words to denote a phrase	`"teenage depression"` will find those documents with these two words appearing together as a phrase
near	Used between two or more search terms or expressions; acts to exclude results based upon proximity. Not available on most search engines.	`teenage near depression` will find those documents with these two words appearing close to one another, which is a broader form of phrase searching
+	Used in front of a word or phrase to denote the word or phrase that must appear in all results	`Freud +Anna` would return only those results that include "Anna"
-	Used in front of a word or phrase to denote the word or phrase that must not appear in any result	`Freud -Anna` would return only those results that did not have "Anna"
Fields ,	Used to specify where to locate your search within each document, in order to increase relevancy of results	`title:depression` will return only those results that have the word "depression" in the document's title. Use `intitle:depression` for Google.

proximity to each of our search items tends to provide us with results of higher relevance.

One such operator is an asterisk *, which acts as a "wildcard symbol." Using it, you can easily find variants to a root term. For "teenage," "teenager," and "teenagers," we can instead specify "`teenag*`." This will find all three variants and cut down on the number of synonyms we need to search under. The wildcard symbol can be combined with any of these other tools to provide greater flexibility.

Other helpful tools are "require" and "exclusion" operators. These are plus and minus signs, respectively: + –, and are similar to the Boolean operators and and not. While not all search engines support this function, you will find it useful with those that do. By placing a plus sign (+) in front of a word (without any spaces between), you can direct the search engine to return only results that include that word. This can be helpful in limiting searches. For example, we may be interested in learning more about Jung's work in psychoanalysis, but not anyone else's. We could, therefore, use a search term such as, psychoanalysis +Jung. This would guarantee that Jung's name will appear in the results, increasing the relevance of our search. In the same way, the minus sign (–) can help you get rid of results which keep showing up which are of no relevance to you. Wanting to learn more about Sigmund Freud via a biography online, for instance, I might want to exclude his daughter, Anna, from the search. Our search term might look like, Freud –Anna. Note that there is no space between the operator and the search term. Some search engines require you use these operators rather than Boolean operators.

The last search tool that will be of use to you is the ability to search only within specific fields. Users of PsycLIT and other commercial databases are undoubtedly accustomed to providing instructions on which field to search in the database. Web search engines, however, tend to be more rudimentary and limit the fields that you can search on. Some of these fields will be of little help to most professionals looking to obtain more relevant results. There is one field, though, which you should become familiar with using. Named the "title:" field, it specifies the title of the Web document and can therefore be useful in trying to find relevant documents. *But beware!* The inclusion of a useful title is solely up to the authors of the document being sought. Many times authors leave specific document titles out (because of space limitations) or have to truncate it severely. So while this may be a good method to try initially, it may restrict your results to too great an extent and will miss many pertinent documents. Fields available for searching are limited to those fields supported by the search engines. A date field, for example, is not available.

Distinguishing Search Engines, Subject Guides, and Meta-Search Engines

There are important differences between a *search engine*, a *subject guide* (or search guide), and a *meta-search engine*. Understanding these differences can make navigating the Web much easier and hassle-free. Search engines are the most popular and widely used ways of searching the Internet for many reasons. First, they are very good at collecting *all* of the data online and indexing it. Second, most provide search tools that allow for relatively easy extraction of that data. Third, there is a wide variety of search engines to choose from, ensuring that individuals are likely to find one that they like the most.

Sometimes search engines, for all of their power and potential, simply don't work well enough. They can still return too many irrelevant results. Also, if you don't know the name of something or the correct term for a subject, a search engine isn't going to help you much. It requires a specific search concept made up of specific keywords.

For these reasons, subject guides (also known as search guides) were developed. They are much like compiled bibliographies or indexes, but they don't rely on software to compile their databases. Instead, they rely on a staff of human editors to search for relevant content online, review it, and place it in their database. This means more of the content will be directly relevant to what you're looking for. It also allows you to find information on a specific topic when you're not sure where to start. You may be able to search *inside* one of these guides. Both search engines and subject guides typically display the results of a search in rank ordering; that is, the most relevant results to your search are displayed first, at the top of the list. As you go further down the list, the relevancy decreases. The downside to guides is that, by definition, they cannot be as comprehensive as a search engine. So you may not be seeing *every* resource listed under a particular subject heading.

Meta-search engines offer you the ability to search across multiple search engines *at the same time*. These meta-search engines also usually offer the ability to intelligently collate the corresponding results, remove duplicate links, check for and remove outdated links or links to online resources that are no longer valid (often referred to as a "bad link"), and then present the results in a rank ordering, with the most relevant results being near the top of the listing.

Other search engines that don't fall neatly into any of the above categories are also becoming available online. One such engine is a piece of software that you download and run from your computer. Much like a meta-search engine, it will send out your search query to a specified set of search engines, collect and collate the results on your desktop. Some of this software may be further specialized to search only certain kinds of databases online, such as those containing only health information. Another search engine that doesn't fall neatly into any category is one that indexes only a few, specialized sites. For example, the American Psychological Association developed PsycCrawler, a search engine that only indexes four or five psychology-oriented Web sites. This was designed to limit the number of irrelevant results returned on a search of the index.

PUTTING THE TOOLS TO USE: DEFINING A SUCCESSFUL SEARCH STRATEGY

How can you successfully and sensibly implement all these search tools? I suggest you think in terms of a *search strategy*. First, you determine whether the type of search you are conducting is one for commonly-available material (e.g., professional resources for the treatment of alcoholism) or more obscure material. If it is a topic that is general and popular, you will have much less difficulty finding it. Beginning in a *subject guide* (also referred to as a *search guide*) is usually the easiest method for this type of search. If you would like to conduct a much more thorough search online, or the material you're seeking is more obscure or specific, you would instead begin with a search engine.

Begin your search by typing in a keyword or two to see how many results you receive. You will probably get quite a few! Then type in the same search phrase using some of the tools listed earlier in the chapter. For example, we could have started off typing in the two words `teenage` and `depression` into the query field. Then we could try placing quotation marks around the terms, such as `"teenage depression"`, or using a Boolean operator such as, `"teenage and depression."` We could also try including all variants of each word and synonyms.

Unfortunately, there is no one or single "correct" way of conducting this search. Why not? Because the type of strategy you will use is determined by the type of search you are conducting. For example, if you'd like to conduct an exhaustive search of all references to Aaron T. Beck online, you may want to use a multitude of keywords, such as `cognitive-behavioral therapy`,`cognitive-behavioral theory`, RET, and `Ellis`. An advanced query on a search engine such as AltaVista might look like

```
Beck and "cognitive behavioral" near (theory or
therapy) and not (RET or Ellis)
```

That is, we want references to Beck, the phrase "cognitive behavioral" near either of the words "theory" or "therapy" and no results returned on either RET (Rational Emotive Therapy) or Ellis (Albert). This isn't really a complete comprehensive search on Beck references online, but it is one of the easiest ways of conducting something close to it (and would be considered a "detailed" search; see Figure 1.1). As you can see, a good query can net you good results.

The single largest problem most people have in searching the Internet is receiving too many irrelevant results. The easiest way to reduce this problem is by typing in more than one keyword, and enclosing words that go together (or phrases) within quotation marks. This simple strategy alone can help narrow your search by over 80% in most cases.

If you take a moment to thoughtfully compose your query using the operators described above, your results will be more rewarding *every time you use a search engine*. This is one of the most important pieces of information you can take away from this book—learn to fully use the power of the search engine you like the best. If you take 5 minutes to read that search engine's help section now, it will save countless hours later of slogging through irrelevant results. As the old computer programming saying goes, "garbage in, garbage out."

What If You Get No Results?

What if your search comes up empty-handed? Usually you will always get *something* in the way of a result when you type in a query. But it's possible, as I've already mentioned, that the information you're seeking simply isn't yet available online. Don't forget: As vast as the Internet is, it still can't com-

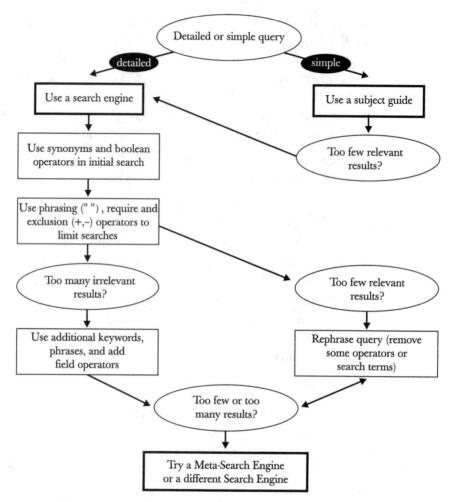

FIGURE 1.1   A simple, general search strategy

pare to the information found in a university's library. Your best strategy when you come up empty-handed is to try rearranging the search terms and use a different combination of operators with different synonyms. If that continues to bring you no relevant results, move on to another search engine. See Chapter 2 for a list of search engines.

A word of caution, however. The Web is still only as good as its current content. Obscure and detailed research topics or highly-specialized and specific subject searches aren't likely to turn up many results no matter what search methodology you use. If you use two or three of the search engines mentioned in the next chapter and keep turning up few results, it's likely that the material you're seeking simply is not available yet online. If your professional area happens to *be* that topic, you could always consider adding to the international knowledge base by putting up your own Web site (which I talk about in Appendix D). Sometimes the library will still be the first and last place to look for information on those kinds of highly-specific topics. By using these search tools, combined with synonyms and an effective search strategy, you will probably be able to find documents on the World Wide Web in a much more time-efficient manner. A summary of the search tools discussed in this chapter is given in Table 1.2.

SECURITY ONLINE

A few years ago, most people connected to the Internet via a telephone line and didn't really have to worry about the security of their home computer. Nowadays, more than 40 million Americans will connect via a broadband connection such as a cable modem or DSL. Many increasingly keep their computers on all the time, because their Internet connection is on all the time and it's just easier than having to wait for the computer to start. But there is a downside to this instant connectivity—the increased security risk to your computer.

Any computer connected to the Internet is susceptible to an attack by a malicious outsider. Traditionally home computers have not been much at risk because their users would log into an Internet service provider through a phone line, and disconnect the moment they finished their online business. The nature of these slow, analog connections made them undesirable targets for a would-be computer attacker. But as home users connect to the Internet via broadband and keep their computers on and online all the time, their home computers now become prime targets for attack. Attackers look for and use home personal computers for larger-scale, coordinated attacks on corporate computer networks, Web sites, and other large targets. Home computers are often much easier to break into because most people's computer settings and operating systems are not very secure.

Entire books have been written about how to create a secure home network and ensure that your personal computer is not subject to an unwanted

TABLE 1.2   Search Engines and the Search Tools They Support

	Operators							
	AND	O R	NOT	Proximity	Phrase	Inclusion/ Exclusion	Wildcard	Field[1]
AltaVista Basic	N/A[2]	default[3]	N/A	N/A	"..."	+ / −	*	host: image: link: text: title: url:
AltaVista Advanced	and/&	or	not	near	"..."	N/A	*	Same
Excite	and	or	and not	N/A	"..."	+ / −	N/A	N/A
AllTheWeb	default	Form-based[4]		N/A	"..."	+ / −	N/A	N/A
Google	default	Form-based[4]		N/A	"..."	+ / −	*	link: site: allintitle: intitle: allinurl: inurl: related: cache:
Hotbot		Form-based[4]		N/A	Advanced search			domain: title:
Lycos		Form-based[4]		N/A	"..."	+ / −	$	N/A
Webcrawler	and	default	not	adj or near	"..."	+ / −	N/A	N/A

Notes:
Different search engines use different combinations of terms to get the same result. For example, Alta-Vista uses just plain not, while Excite requires the words and not to be used instead. Within individual search engines, they may also allow different operators to get the same result (e.g., AltaVista allows you to use either and or the ampersand symbol (&) to specify the Boolean term and).

[1]Field—Search engines may allow searching on technical fields such as anchor, applet, or host, which are not relevant for most readers.

[2]N/A—Not applicable. This operator is not supported by this search engine.

[3]Default—This is the default operator used when you type in two words together. For example, "teenage depression" will be searched for as "teenage or depression" in AltaVista, but Open Text will interpret the query as "teenage and depression."

[4]Form-based—Uses a specialized form you fill out on their Web site in order to specify these options.

attack. Each operating system is different (even among versions of Microsoft Windows), so it is difficult to suggest security methods here that will work for everyone. I will make the following general recommendations, however, that will give you a place to start:

■ **If you are a cable or DSL user, invest in either a software or hardware "firewall."** A firewall is either a piece of software or a small hardware device that basically acts as a traffic cop between your computer (or your home computer network) and the Internet. It examines all communications coming into your computer or network, as well as all communications going out to the Internet. It checks the technical format of these communications to ensure they are expected. Unexpected or known attacker communications are forbidden and turned away. It prevents your computer from being used as a means of launching a larger attack against some other computer as well. Best of all, software firewalls can be found for free online. Zone Labs makes a free version of its firewall, called ZoneAlarm, available through its Web site at http://www.zonelabs.com/. Hardware solutions often come in the form of cable/DSL routers, such as those made by Linksys (http://www.linksys.com/) or Netgear (http://www.netgear.com/). Their products can often be found in large electronics retailers as well.

■ **Install virus software.** Nearly all new computers manufactured today provide free trial subscriptions to anti-virus software. These often require an annual paid subscription when the trial runs out. Such software can help protect most average Internet users from the malicious viruses that often circulate online. An alternative to such programs is GRISOFT's free AVG AntiVirus Free Edition. Their virus software is just as good as the commercial versions and is available from their Web site at http://www.grisoft.com/.

■ **Use ShieldsUP!** Gibson Research Corporation has made an interesting security diagnostic tool, called ShieldsUP!, available for free on its Web site at http://grc.com/default.htm. This tool will examine your computer's Internet connection and settings and determine whether any of them should be of concern. It will then guide you through steps to make your computer more secure. This free tool has been accessed over 20 million times and is a safe, quick way to determine whether your computer is vulnerable to Internet attacks. Consider its recommendations seriously.

■ **Turn your computer off.** Most modern computers nowadays can start in a much shorter time span than did those of 5 or 10 years ago. If you use your computer infrequently, or just once a day, it's likely worth the short additional wait in order to keep your computer much more secure. The security you gain from simply shutting your computer off is hard to match.

■ **Do not click on e-mail attachments directly or install software you did not request.** In this day and age, it is difficult not to get e-mail that has attachments. Colleagues send word processing documents back and forth through e-mail daily, family members send digital pictures of loved ones, and your friend wants you to take a look at the latest home digital video he made. These are examples of e-mail attachments that are okay to click on, because you know the sender and were expecting something from them. When an unexpected or cryptic e-mail comes to you, however, *do not* automatically click on the attachment. Some e-mail viruses cleverly disguise themselves as friendly attachments that unsuspecting users automatically click on without thinking twice. Double-check with the e-mail sender first to ensure they did indeed send you a legitimate attachment. If the sender is unknown to you, the safest thing to do is delete the e-mail and the attachment—without opening them—immediately.

E-mail from unrecognized or unfamiliar names with attachments is nearly always spam and can be discarded without a second thought. Most virus programs will also detect a virus masquerading as a legitimate e-mail attachment and disable or delete it long before it causes your computer any harm (assuming you have virus software running!). Unlike paper documents, a deleted legitimate e-mail can readily be replaced by asking the sender to resend it.

With the explosion of advertising online, some may try to get you to install some piece of software on your computer. It may be advertised as software that will speed up your Internet connection, or make your computer more secure. (If you followed the previous recommendations, your computer is already secure enough!) Unless you need the software in order to complete a specific task related to that particular Web site, I would highly recommend forgoing installation of unrequested software on your computer. Most such software is actually advertising and marketing software in disguise. This kind of software, called "spyware" or "adware," is specifically designed to monitor your online activities and report back to the marketing and advertising companies where you go and what you search for online. They sell this data to other companies, who then market specific products to you through numerous new pop-up advertising on your computer. Unless you enjoy more advertising during your online experience, I would suggest staying away from any advertisement online that requests your permission to install software.

2

Knowing Where to Look Online

Now that you've got the tools and the search strategy down, where do you go to employ them online? You can use these tools at many of the Web sites listed in Part II of this book. But every day new materials and sites come online. How can you be sure to stay current? This chapter tells you how. But first, let me mention where *not* to start looking online.

People often start their online searches by simply typing something into their Web browser's address box. While this may work as a quick-and-dirty search technique, it is not the best way to conduct a useful online search. This type of search uses the Web browser's default search engine, which is often not the best search engine available.

Your choice of search tools should be based upon a number of factors. One factor is the quality and size of its database. Larger search engines tend to be better for more advanced or rigorous searches, but smaller databases can sometimes be useful. A second factor is the query tools available to you from the search engine. Although most people are familiar with typing in one or two keywords into a search box, they do not know that there are often more advanced and richer tools available to them under the "Advanced Search" option, or by simply reading the search engine's help file. These options vary from tool to tool. Becoming familiar with these tools and the advanced options available will lead to better, more relevant search results.

The third, and perhaps most important factor, is choosing the right search tool for the right kind of job. Typing in a general term such as "free Web hosting" into almost any search engine will give you thousands of virtually useless results if you are just looking for a site to host your Web page for free. Typing the same term into a directory or subject guide, such as Yahoo! or the Open Directory Project, however, will lead you to categories that contain just those few dozen sites of relevance, with very little trouble. How do you know when to use a directory instead of a search engine? If typing in additional keywords and phrases into a search engine doesn't help refine and narrow your search results, try a subject guide or directory instead. (Note that you can, however, change this default in both Netscape and Microsoft browsers. Newer versions of Netscape and Microsoft

UNDERSTANDING WEB RESOURCE HEADINGS AND THE RATING SYSTEM

In most sections of this book, World Wide Web resources are listed in alphabetical order by their respective names or what I refer to as "titles." The "owner" of the resource is then noted. The owner is the person or organization responsible for the Web site, its ongoing maintenance and most importantly, its content. Listed next is the Web resource's address online, also known as its *uniform resource locator* or URL. Additional URLs, which point to a specific resource described within the narrative or if two services reside on the same site, may be listed. A rating and narrative review of each site summarizes the highlights and downsides of the site.

The system I use throughout this book to rate Web sites is based on those commonly used by other online rating services. Ratings take into consideration four central quality categories:

■ *Content*—Does the site add *new and unique* material to the online world, or does it simply list or link to existing material well covered by other sites already? Does it offer new insights or offer information not found elsewhere? Does it offer refreshing perspectives, and/or regularly updated new content in the form of news articles, opinions, or other forms of communication? Does it include interactive features? Is it just an advertisement for an organization or company? Is it objective and fair? Does it present misinformation or common popular fallacies?

■ *Presentation*–Is the information laid out in a logical and well-organized manner? Are graphics designed appropriately for the site and do they appear on your computer quickly? Do the graphics overwhelm the user and the content? Is it arranged so the best material the site has to offer is clearly delineated from other, less-important material?

■ *Ease-of-use*–Can you find your way to particular content quickly using the navigation aids provided, and then get back to where you entered the Web site just as easily? Is the *user interface* (the means by which the Web site interacts with you) well designed? Are a search engine or other tools provided to help a person find information more quickly (when appropriate)? Can you easily find an e-mail address on the page to provide feedback about broken links or the like?

■ *Overall experience*–What kind of feelings did I have when I came away from the site? Was it enjoyable or painful to read? Was I expecting more and became disappointed by the content or presentation or difficulty in navigating through the site? Would I *bookmark* (add it to my "bookmark" or "favorite places" list in my Web browser) the site myself or find myself wanting to return on a regular basis?

A four-star system is used to denote the result of ratings in these categories:

■ ★★★★–*Excellent.* One of the best sites on the Web for this topic due to its outstanding design and content.

■ ★★★–*Very good.* Worth your time to visit. Well designed with robust and useful content.

■ ★★–*Average.* A solid online resource filled with basic but generally uninteresting information.

■ ★–*Poor.* Lacking important content or difficult to use.

Please note that a site may obtain different ratings throughout the book depending on the category under which it is being rated. The American Psychological Association's PsychNET Web site, for example, is an excellent professional association site (rating four stars), but a less-interesting consumer resources site (rating only three stars).

browsers also have search windows or sidebars that open up on the side of the browser window. In the sidebar, a user can conduct a more advanced search and even choose which search engine they want to query. This is a helpful shortcut for advanced users, because it cuts out the step of actually having to visit the search engine's homepage to begin.)

This chapter presents a list of the larger and more popular search engines, subject guides and directories, and meta-search engines online today. Although this list is not comprehensive, it does give you a broad selection of what's available, along with brief descriptions and reviews of their abilities. Those listed tend to have a record of stability and are therefore likely to be around for a long time. I'll also discuss other methods for finding information that go beyond simple Web searches (such as utilizing newsgroups and mailing lists). I will discuss the pros and cons of each method for searching and tell you what kind of searches are best for each method. Before going on to this list, you should take a look at the box explaining the list's format and the rating system I have used for each resource.

THE FIRST CHOICE FOR DETAILED QUESTIONS: SEARCH ENGINES

All search engines use automated software (referred to as Web "crawlers," "spiders," or "robots") to compile their databases. This software is generally very good at finding information on the Internet and storing it within an index. The numbers bandied about to claim each is the "largest and most comprehensive" database online are largely meaningless. All such databases are pretty much similar in size. Size, here anyway, doesn't really matter. What is important is the flexibility and power of the retrieval software. If a search engine has a large database, but the tools for extracting information from it are rudimentary, it's not going to be all that useful. On the other hand, a large database combined with excellent tools make for a winning combination. The key to those tools, though, is knowing that they exist, learning how to use them effectively, and having them work as they were intended to work.

None of the currently available search engines remove duplicate results. Most also have difficulty in discriminating among results that point to the slightly different pages of the same Web site. This means that you could view a search engine's results of four or five pages, all of which lead to the same Web site! This may not be a bad thing if all the pages are relevant to your search topic, but more often than not, that is not the case.

Companies have been experimenting for years now on how best to integrate advertising with search results. The highly rated Google includes advertising in its search results. It does this with unobtrusive text advertising to the right of the search results, with no more than two advertisements displayed above the search results. To ensure there's no confusion that these two advertisements are not actual search results, they are further set off with different-colored backgrounds. This helps to clearly distinguish advertising from search results provided by Google's unique search algorithm, while also not interfering with the display of the most relevant, free results.

Overture is the latest player in the online search advertising game, and it has acquired some recognizable veteran search engines to help its cause. This advertising company owns both AltaVista.com and AllTheWeb.com, and they have stated they will use both Web sites to test new advertising methods. Overture's traditional advertising method in search engines is to offer paid-placement advertising directly above the search engine results. These results often look just like the actual search engine's results and are sometimes delineated with nothing but very small text indicating that they are sponsored ads. The simple deception is more effective than you might think. Naive users often will click on the first few links presented in a search engine's results without paying attention to the tiny print. You can readily see this in action at a site such as Search.com (reviewed in the meta-search section below) or portal site MSN.com.

The largest obstacle facing advertising networks such as Overture is how to present advertising in a way that isn't likely to dissuade most users from using theirs and others' search engines. As Internet users become aware of these deceptive advertising methods, they will turn away from their default search engines and turn to search engines that offer not only the most relevant results, but also present advertising in a direct, nondeceptive manner.

If you would like to keep updated on the latest developments in the world of online search engines, you should regularly visit the premier site for this information: `http://www.searchenginewatch.com/`.

The Most Popular, Useful, and Widely Used Search Engines

There are dozens of search engines available for searching the Web. Only a handful of them, however, are widely used because of their ability to provide reliable access to their large databases. Search engines are the most-often visited Web sites online, so being able to reach them is an important factor to consider. All of the engines listed below are stable online resources with similarly large databases, which are updated daily. They differ mainly in their ability to provide relevant results. They are listed alphabetically.

Title (or descriptor):	AltaVista
Owner:	Overture
URL (Web address):	`http://www.altavista.com/`
Rating:	★★★

AltaVista was once one of the most powerful and widely used search engines, for good reason. It still offers a large database and the most powerful and flexible retrieval tools available. AltaVista offers one of two types of searching: "Basic" and "Advanced." Basic searching is the default and is often adequate. One of AltaVista's quirks is that when using "Basic" searching, you cannot use Boolean operators (such as `and`, `or`, and `not`) or the `near` operator. To use these options, you must choose "Advanced" searching. Use the advanced option to conduct a serious AltaVista search on the Internet.

AltaVista also offers the ability to search the Internet by specific fields within each Web document. Every document on the Web, much like every page in a book, is displayed in a visual format defined by hidden formatting codes. By searching within these specific codes, or fields, you can further limit your search and help increase relevancy. In AltaVista you can use this option combined with other operators and options, and it can be used within a basic or advanced search. One example of utilizing this feature would be to limit your search only to the title field of the document. For instance:

```
title:freud
```

Note that there is a colon but *no space* between the field you wish to search and the search term itself. This would greatly limit your search, since only those files that had the term "freud" *in their title* (capitalization here is unimportant) would be returned. I received about 20,000 documents using this method as opposed to just typing in "freud," which returned over 425,000 results from AltaVista! Using this method is no guarantee of increasing relevancy; it will exclude perfectly relevant and useful documents that simply don't have the keyword in the title. But it can be helpful when used sparingly or to narrow your search.

Another helpful tool in the AltaVista search arsenal is the ability to browse through a directory of Web sites. Many search engines have incorporated directory browsing (popularized by Yahoo!) as an alternative method for finding information online. AltaVista's directory is actually powered by LookSmart (see entry in next section). In addition to searching ordinary documents online, AltaVista also allows searches for images, music and video files, and news, among other options. It has thankfully scaled back its ambitions in recent years to become a central portal destination and is once again focusing on its search technologies. AltaVista's innovative BabelFish, an automated language translation technology, is also a well-known and useful tool.

A newer feature of AltaVista is AltaVista Prisma. Prisma provides additional phrases directly related to your search query at the top of your search results. When you click on one of these phrases, AltaVista provides a more refined search. In theory, this is a good idea for helping you to pare down your searches, but in practice, it doesn't always offer helpful phrases relevant to your search.

Since its acquisition by Overture, however, AltaVista has suffered from advertising result overload. Its search results are now peppered with so many advertisements (labeled "Sponsored Matches") appearing before the actual results that it is a little overwhelming and ridiculous. AltaVista deserves an even lower rating, were it not for the great set of helpful tools offered by the site.

Title (or descriptor):	AllTheWeb
Owner:	Overture
URL (Web address):	`http://www.alltheweb.com/`
Rating:	★★★

AllTheWeb is a newer generation of search engine that, like AltaVista, allows searches not only on plain Web documents, but also on images and audio and video files. With one of the largest indexes on the Internet, and with few irrelevant results, it is a reliable, quick, and powerful site to run your searches on. Its advanced form is a powerful tool to create more complex queries.

Since being acquired by Overture, AllTheWeb has suffered the same decline in quality as AltaVista, but to a lesser extent as of this writing. Some sponsored ads are offered in search results, but the ads tend to be fewer and identified by a small "Sponsored" notation. Unexpectedly, I found AltaVista's older search algorithm to be slightly superior to AllTheWeb's newer and larger one, which tended to present fewer relevant results.

Title (or descriptor):	Ask Jeeves
Owner:	Ask Jeeves, Inc.
URL (Web address):	`http://www.ask.com/`
Rating:	★★

This search engine was once assembled by human editors that carefully reviewed each entry included within its database. Now that the World Wide Web consists of billions of pages and hundreds of millions of sites, that is no longer the case. Search results can be relevant, but it really depends on the type of query. Ask Jeeve's natural language querying ability—you can type in a question in everyday English—is more of a marketing ploy than a useful feature given people's wide exposure to Internet searching. The most frustrating component that will likely contribute to the site's stagnation is the fee requirement in order to submit a new Web site to its index. Nearly ever other search engine on the Web (except its corporate sister, Teoma) requires no such fee. A submission fee becomes an obstacle for most personal and smaller independent sites, and its database will likely eventually become skewed by commercial interests.

Title (or descriptor):	Enpsychlopedia
Owner:	PsychCentral.com
URL (Web address):	`http://enpsychlopedia.com/`
Rating:	★★

A specialized search engine, focused only on a dozen or so mental health and psychology Web sites (including PsychCentral.com, a site I own and maintain), this search engine has some potential. With the growth of the Internet, it is becoming increasingly difficult for general search engines, even those as good as Google, to return results that are not full of the irrelevant advertisements or pharmaceutical-backed sites. Enpsychlopedia with its clean, Google-like interface, is an attempt to return quality search results no matter what, because it indexes only a few relevant mental health and psychology sites. If it was faster and provided a somewhat larger index, it would be more useful. As it is today, it may be too small to be of much use to professionals.

Google

Title (or descriptor):	Google
Owner:	Google, Inc.
URL (Web address):	`http://www.google.com/`
Rating:	★★★★

Google is the premier innovative search engine in a field that was in need of some innovation. The relevancy of results returned is determined by a number of factors. Not only does it search for keywords within the pages it indexes, but it also uses proximity of those words to one another, and the number of other pages that link to each document to formulate a complex relevancy equation. The outcome of this equation is that results returned are usually more relevant than those returned by other search engines. With an index of more than 3 billion Web pages, Google is by far the largest index on the Internet today. This size makes searches about as comprehensive as can be obtained, leading some to consider Google the gold standard for searching the Internet.

Like AOL Search and some other search engines, Google offers a browsable directory of Web sites (the same index maintained by the Open Directory Project, below), searches on specific fields of a Web document, such as its title or in links found within a document, as well as on images. A unique feature of Google unavailable on other search engines is its page cache. Not only has Google indexed more than 3 billion Web pages, it also stores a copy of them on its own servers. This allows a user to access the page's content even when it has been removed from the original site, or if the original site is temporarily (or permanently) unavailable.

Google is also home of the old Usenet Internet newsgroup archive, Deja.com, now called Google Groups. This service allows Web-based access to these interactive discussion forums. The archive holds over a terabyte of information, with more than 650 million individual messages dating back to 1995.

What is really very striking about Google's search technique, compared with other search engines on the Internet today, is how well it filters out the "noise" that often intrudes into otherwise relevant results. It's not foolproof and can still be tricked by search engine optimization techniques used by some Web developers, which seek to have their sites score higher in a result listing than they legitimately should. But Google's engineers are constantly updating and attempting to improve their search algorithm—a level of maintenance sorely missing from other search engines. At least twice a year, Google engineers change the search algorithm to discourage these search engine optimization techniques and to improve the relevancy of results. It is this attention to detail that keeps Google on top.

ADVERTISING ONLINE

Advertising online is now as commonplace as it is on television. Most of the advertising is generally innocuous—a small graphic that runs at the top or on the side of each page. On search engines, however, there may be more at work to produce that ad than meets the eye. Using an advertising technique called "targeted marketing," search engines display advertisements directly related to the search terms entered. For example, if you enter the term, "computer buying" into a search engine, you might receive an advertisement on the search results page for a computer maker, such as Gateway or Dell.

Another trend in online advertising is a change in how advertisers pay for their ads. Traditionally, advertisers paid Web developers based upon how many times their ad was shown on a page. More and more advertisers are backing away from this business model, however, and are moving toward paying based upon the number of people who actually click on the ad. A "click-through," as they are called, means a person is more likely interested in the product or service being sold. But since click-throughs account for only 1–2% of the people who actually see the ad, advertisers and developers are working on still more intrusive strategies to increase advertising revenue and sales. One such strategy used to try and enhance people's interest in a product or service is to make the advertisement nearly indistinguishable from editorial content on the Web site. This type of online advertising is another disturbing trend which will hopefully be short-lived. When content becomes blurred with advertising in this manner, the usefulness of the online world as an information medium diminishes substantially. Yet another form of online revenue generation is an "association" with a book or music retailer. These associations return 5–25% of any purchases made online through them to the Web site's owner.

Unlike most other search engines, Google provides direct access to its huge Internet database to Web developers through a programming interface. This allows enterprising developers to build their own tools for searching Google, an interesting way to encourage creative development from outside programmers that might otherwise not occur. To date, hundreds of such tools have been built. This has led other Internet heavyweights, such as Amazon.com, to begin offering similar functionality to their databases.

Google's advanced operators also allow searching on titles (`allintitle`), URLs (`allinurl`), and domains (`site`). Using such operators can help you greatly refine your search. For example, to search for only the words "Sigmund Freud" in the title, you could type:

```
allintitle:Sigmund Freud
```

This will return results of all documents with both of the words, Sigmund and Freud in the title of the Web document. If you only want to find results for a search query from a particular Web site, for instance, WebMD.com, you would type:

```
site:webmd.com sigmund freud
```

This search would return only those documents from WebMD.com that mention Sigmund Freud.

Title (or descriptor):	HotBot
Owner:	Lycos, Inc.
URL (Web address):	`http://www.hotbot.com/`
Rating:	★★

HotBot is one of the few remaining search engines available that provides a clean, simple interface and the ability to search the Inktomi-developed database. Inktomi is a search engine developer that has been around a long time but was acquired in 2003 by Yahoo! Oddly, HotBot also allows separate searches on other databases, including Google, Teoma, and AllTheWeb. HotBot supports the use of Boolean operators and phrases, as well as a number of other unique search tools. These include the ability to search by the date a particular Web page was indexed by the search engine, the type of media (e.g., if you're searching for an audio file or particular image), among others. As with nearly all search engine providers today, the first couple of results were sponsored links (noted by a small, difficult-to-read "sponsored link" notation), followed by the actual search engine results. Additional text advertisements can be seen along the right-hand side of the results, à la Google.

Title (or descriptor):   Lycos
Owner: Lycos, Inc.
URL (Web address):   http://www.lycos.com/
Rating: ★

Lycos is one of the oldest and most well-known search engines online, but it has fallen into virtual obscurity, having been surpassed by tools far better suited for most users' tasks. Its results, although usually relevant, are more susceptible than other engines to developer's tricks to get their Web sites listed closer to the top of a results page. The results pages themselves are cluttered with too much advertising. Lycos uses the Open Directory Project (see next section) to offer users a browseable directory of sites. This search engine has seen better days; its current incarnation is a hollow shell for one of the pioneers in this online area.

SCIrUS
for scientific information only

Title (or descriptor):   Scirus
Owner: Elsevier Science
URL (Web address):   http://www.scirus.com/
Rating: ★★★★

Scirus came on the scene of specialized search engines a few years ago and appears to have finally come into its own. Using the same database as developed for the AlltheWeb.com search engine, it claims to focus only on Web sites that provide scientific content. It can read nontext files, search databases such as MEDLINE, and can more easily locate peer-reviewed articles than can traditional search engines. In my tests, it lived up to its claims. It consistently returned higher quality results than did the same queries run on general Internet search engines, such as Google. It has minimal advertising and lets you sort your results by either relevance or by date. Scirus also lets you save your search preferences, and an advanced search page, which gives you precise control over what databases and content stores are searched, is available. One thing to note about specialized search engines such as Scirus is that by their very nature, they tend not to be as inclusive as a general search engine. I don't think this is a drawback, however, when the growth of the Internet continues at its current astounding rate.

Title (or descriptor):	Teoma
Owner:	Ask Jeeves, Inc.
URL (Web address):	`http://www.teoma.com/`
Rating:	★★

Teoma is one of the newer search engines, owned by the same company that offers Ask Jeeves. Trying to combat the problem of irrelevant search results, Teoma provides two additional components to each results page: refine and resources. Refine provides additional phrases related to your search query, much like AltaVista's Prisma feature does. A good idea, but in practice, all it does is add those keywords to your search. (Teoma doesn't even bother treating the words as a phrase to help refine your search.) This appears to be a poor attempt at refining. Resources are supposed to be sites that are authoritative sources for additional links on the query topic. Unfortunately, this Teoma component cannot really distinguish an authoritative source from a regular Web site, and often lists both in this category. Without providing a reliable ability to distinguish between the two, Teoma's resource component also is fairly useless. Teoma provides sponsored results at the top of regular results in an area with a different color background than regular results, helping to distinguish them. Like its corporate sister, Ask Jeeves, Teoma only accepts site submissions to its index if the site is willing to pay its submission fee. This makes Teoma a search engine likely to be biased in the future toward commercial sites and others that are willing and can afford to pay the fee.

ASSEMBLED BY HUMAN HANDS: SUBJECT/SEARCH GUIDES AND DIRECTORIES

As discussed earlier (see Chapter 1) subject or search guides rely on human editors rather than software to find information on the Internet and index it. There are two primary types of search guides: general and specific. General guides act like a library's card catalog organized by broad subjects. They cover everything under the sun, from computers to entertainment, from hobbies to psychology, from cars to clothing, and a whole lot more. The specific guides limit themselves to particular online topic areas. So there might be a guide to psychology online, or neuropsychology, or depression.

These latter types of guides tend to be smaller, by definition, but more comprehensive within the subject they cover than the general-purpose guides. Both types of these guides are included in the alphabetical list below.

Title (or descriptor):	healthfinder™
Owner:	U.S. Department of Health and Human Services
URL (Web address):	`http://www.healthfinder.gov/`
Rating:	★★★★

This informative and extensive search guide from the U.S. Department of Health and Human Services offers links to health and mental health information found on hundreds of Web sites, but most of them are overseen by the U.S. federal government. The site has grown considerablly since its inception, and continues to improve weekly. This site is unique in that it not only provides you with the usual hypertext links to other sites, but in many cases to their real-world contact information, such as phone numbers and addresses. Descriptions are brief but helpful and the site has a simple yet effective design.

Title (or descriptor):	Medical Matrix
Owner:	Medical Matrix, LLC
URL (Web address):	
	`http://www.medmatrix.org/_SPages/Psychiatry.asp`
Rating:	★★

Updated regularly, this is a peer-reviewed guide to a wide variety of medical resources online, including a section devoted to psychiatry. Each subcategory is arranged by Medical Subject Headings (MeSH), a medical standard for arranging information developed by the U.S. National Library of Medicine, and includes news, abstracts, reviews, articles, meeting reports, major resources, indices, reference documents, learning modules, practice guidelines, cases meetings, textbooks, diseases, forums, and patient education. Listings are relatively short and incomplete, and some were quite out-of-date. An internal search engine and logical layout of resources make navigation through the Matrix a breeze. Good for use mainly as a quick-start guide to the world of online medical resources. Requires an $89 annual subscription fee in order to gain access, but a 24-hour free pass is available for new users.

Title (or descriptor):	Mental Help Net
Owner:	Centersite, LLC
URL (Web address):	`http://mentalhelp.net/`
Rating:	★★★

Mental Help Net is an example of a field-specific search guide that I cofounded. It covers resources only within the mental health, psychological, and psychiatric fields. Because it limits itself to those professions and is maintained by a staff of professionals, it can be quite good about maintaining a comprehensive catalog of relevant resources. Unlike general-purpose guides, Mental Help Net offers large listings of professional and lay resources online in specific subcategories (e.g., cognitive, assessment, psychopharmacology, etc.) and disorders (e.g., major depression, anxiety, PTSD, etc.). Like other guides, it also has an internal search engine that searches within the Web site, to make it easier to find topics quickly. Mental Help Net uses a unique combination of software, human editors, and reader feedback to find, rate, and review the resources found within its database.

Like many other Internet directories, Mental Help Net reviews and provides a rating for Internet resources in mental health and psychology. In recent years, however, its database of these resources has become outdated, inaccurate, and full of dead links to nowhere. New reviews of Internet resources appear to be added rarely. A number of additional databases are available on the site, including one that keeps track of the over 1,600 journal Web sites online. The Web site's more recent attempts at advertising and branding have been confusing and less successful.

Title (or descriptor):	Online Dictionary of Mental Health
Owner:	Centre for Psychotherapeutic Studies, University of Sheffield
URL (Web address):	`http://www.human-nature.com/odmh/`
Rating:	★★

This is an eclectic offering from the Centre for Psychotherapeutic Studies, incorporating both the *Online Dictionary of Mental Health* and the *Online Dictionary of Ideas*. Basically replicating guides and resources already found on the Web, this guide allows both alphabetical and subject browsing and provides an internal search engine. Descriptions for many resources are provided. Nothing stands out about this resource except its unique inclusion of links to information and resources on philosophers and thinkers throughout history (through its *Online Dictionary of Ideas*). Some of its graphics seem amateurish and less than obvious in their meaning. North American users may find the site slow to load since it is located in the United Kingdom; European users will appreciate the site's proximity, however. The Guide to Psychotherapy is easy to navigate and logically arranged. Infrequently updated.

Title (or descriptor):	Open Directory Project
Owner:	Netscape
URL (Web address):	http://www.dmoz.org/
Rating:	★★★★

Billing itself as the "largest human-edited directory of the Web," it's not hard to see how it lives up to its reputation—over 58,000 of its volunteer editors are keeping track of over 4 million sites that the directory indexes in over 460,000 categories. This is far more than the hundreds of editors Yahoo! employs, and ideally, leads not only to more diversity in the sites listed, but ultimately more sites listed. The volunteer editors only manage categories in which they are experienced. Because of its open, noncommercial nature, the Open Directory Project has the potential to be one of the largest and most interesting collaborative online projects in history. It has the best chance of being able to keep up with the Internet's enormous growth.

Title (or descriptor):	Psych Web
Owner:	Russell A. Dewey, PhD
URL (Web address):	http://www.psychwww.com/
Rating:	★★★

Located in Georgia Southern University's Psychology Department, Russell Dewey developed one of the older and more popular online guides to mental health and psychology. Arranged in a topical hierarchy, resources are generally easy to find although an internal search engine for a site of this size would be appreciated. Unique contributions to the online world include the complete text of two classics, *The Interpretation of Dreams* (3rd edition) by Sigmund Freud and *Varieties of Religious Experience* by William James. The site not only hosts a wide variety of professional and lay resources, but also includes specific categories for psychology students, links to brochures and articles in psychology, and a psychology of religion section.

Title (or descriptor):	Yahoo!
Owner:	Yahoo!, Inc.
URL (Web address):	`http://www.yahoo.com/`
Rating:	★★★★

Easily the most popular and well known of the search guides, Yahoo! is also one of the oldest search methods available online. While Yahoo! is better known than the Open Directory Project, it indexes fewer resources and takes much longer for new sites to be included in its database (if at all). The reason Yahoo! has remained popular is its ease-of-use, simple and fast-loading pages, and its reputation. Yahoo! staffers review each site listed, and award a set of sunglasses (considered one of the premier online awards) to the sites they deem the best. Yahoo! reviews Web sites for inclusion or exclusion within its catalog, but it doesn't provide actual reviews to sites it indexes. It relies on the individuals who submit their Web sites to provide a short, one-line description to include with their site if it ends up being listed in Yahoo!. Yahoo!'s criteria for inclusion into its guide are unclear, and some Web developers of perfectly good sites complain of not being included. But for an easy-to-navigate, general-purpose subject guide, this is still the best and largest online today. Even professionals will find much to explore on this site, which also offers the ability to customize your own search method. This allows you to receive personalized news summaries, sports scores, and other tidbits.

DOING THE LEGWORK FOR YOU: META-SEARCH ENGINES

The last category covered in this chapter is perhaps one of the most interesting developments online today and a portent of the future. Meta-search engines offer the ability to send a search query across all the search engines previously listed. The meta-search engine then intelligently collates the results, removing duplicatons and broken links. The downside to this wonderful technology is long wait times. Some search sites on the Web are more popular (and therefore slower to respond) than others. It can also be difficult at times to access the meta-search engine Web site itself, since these are becoming increasingly popular as they become better known among Web users.

Just because you're searching six or eight search engines at the same time doesn't mean you're more likely to get more relevant results, either. You're just saving yourself the hassle of having to visit the six Web sites yourself and do the same search six times. However, it is sometimes more productive to visit the sites individually because of the lack of uniformity of search tools of each engine. Meta-search engines can't be as specific or as powerful in their searches because not every search engine understands the same syntax (as discussed earlier).

One other caveat about these types of search engines. Some of them listed below may be somewhat experimental. While I have made every attempt to verify their existence and stability, by the time this book is published, some of these may have been superseded by others.

Title (or descriptor):	CNET Search.com
Owner:	CNET Networks, Inc.
URL (Web address):	http://www.search.com/
Rating:	★★

Having acquired the SavvySearch technology in 2000, CNET's Search.com now uses the same technology to power its metasearch engine. Like other metasearch engines, Search.com simultaneously sends your query to multiple Internet search engines (including About.com, AltaVista, AskJeeves, FindWhat, LookSmart, the Open Directory Project, Sprinks, Surf Point, Thunderstone, and Yahoo!) and returns a complete set of rank-ordered results. This site allows you to customize which search engines and other resources it queries, and it can remember your preferences upon your return. For instance, if you'd rather not receive any results from Find-What.com, simply uncheck that box in the Advanced search area. Many of the search databases that Search.com relies on are themselves fairly unreliable in providing relevant results. If you are going to use Search.com on a regular basis, you should go to the Advanced Settings page and uncheck Search Sponsors and Latest Prices (unless these categories are of specific interest to you), and check Web Pages and Directories. By doing this, your search results will not contain the usual large section of sponsored links that appear before the actual search results. The ability of Search.com to provide even a single page of completely relevant results, however, is still often taxed.

Title (or descriptor):	Excite
Owner:	Focus Interactive, Inc.
URL (Web address):	`http://www.excite.com/`
Rating:	★

Once one of the stars of the dot.com boom in the late 1990s, Excite has turned into a useless search engine providing more advertising to users than any other search engine or Web portal I know of. Search results are nearly 80% sponsored results, with so little distinction made between the results that are sponsored and those that are not as to be purposely confusing to the user. Getting its actual search data from InfoSpace, Inc., a provider of search engine results from multiple databases, Excite no longer even maintains its own search data. Whereas once this search engine had a small following of older Internet users, I cannot imagine a reason for ever visiting it today.

Title (or descriptor):	MetaCrawler
Owner:	InfoSpace, Inc.
URL (Web address):	`http://www.metacrawler.com/`
Rating:	★

Metacrawler, owned and powered by InfoSpace's search technology, offers search results from six different search engines. Few of these engines, however, offer the kind of quality that one has come to expect from an online search engine solution, such as Google. Results are peppered with irrelevant Web sites that have used search engine optimization techniques to artificially inflate their rankings. InfoSpace has done a good job of either purchasing or providing the search engine results for many of the search engines reviewed here. Unfortunately, its search engine technology is a generation or two behind the leaders.

Title (or descriptor):   ProFusion

Owner: Intelliseek, Inc.

URL (Web address):   http://www.profusion.com/

Rating: ★★★

ProFusion is a meta-search engine designed to showcase the technology behind it. It searches "one thousand sources of authoritative information," but doesn't tell the user which "one thousand" specific sources it uses. It uniquely offers a search of the so-called "invisible Web," documents that traditionally have not been indexed by search engines (such as PDF files or online databases). ProFusion also allows the user to limit the search to specific search engines (it currently searches AOL, Lycos, AltaVista, Teoma, Overture, and Yahoo!), but some of these use the same search database.

Title (or descriptor):   SuperSearch III

Owner: Robert Olsson

URL (Web address):   http://www.robtex.com/search.htm

Rating: ★★

This is not a true meta-search engine, but rather a simple interface to shuttle your query to a number of search engines simultaneously. SuperSearch III doesn't limit you to just two or three search engines, but has over a dozen to choose from. It suffers from drawbacks, however, including extremely slow loading time of results (because of the graphics on each search engine's results page). It displays the results of each engine in tiny frames on one page. Needless to say, while it may be useful on a rare occasion, it is likely to be more annoying than helpful. Because it utilizes both frames and Javascript, you'll need a Javascript- and frames-enabled browser.

Title (or descriptor):   Vivisimo

Owner: Vivisimo, Inc.

URL (Web address):   http://www.vivisimo.com/

Rating: ★★★

Vivisimo is a new type of metasearch engine that uses a proprietary algorithm to produce *document clusters,* which help improve the relevancy of results returned. Vivisimo has the ability to group similarly related documents into folders, and it searches nine of the most popular search engines and directories (currently including Lycos, Netscape, LookSmart, and MSN), removes likely duplicates, and returns 200 results at a time. Vivisimo's meta-search engine is a technology demonstration for its unique search software.

Title (or descriptor):	Webcrawler
Owner:	Infospace, Inc.
URL (Web address):	`http://www.webcrawler.com/`
Rating:	★

Webcrawler is one of the oldest search engines online and the first to index the full text of each Web page in its database. Unfortunately, due to its inability to keep up with its tremendous growth since 1995, it has fallen behind both technologically and in the smallish size of its database.

MetaCrawler, like many other generic search engines such as Excite, now gets its search data from multiple search databases provided by its most recent owner, InfoSpace, Inc. This means that sponsored results are interspersed with nonsponsored (or real search results), and on Webcrawler, they do not differentiate between the two. There is no reason to use this search engine.

HOW TO FIND AND SEARCH DISCUSSION FORUMS: MAILING LISTS AND USENET NEWSGROUPS

There is no inherent advantage to searching for information in newsgroups or mailing lists, since most of these forums are simply ongoing conversations among many people. But you can use this type of search in a unique way. For example, you could search for individuals discussing a particular topic to find out where to go to join in on the discussion. Or you might use these tools to find another professional somewhere in the world who's interested in the same research questions (or clinical topics) as you are. Anything that anybody has ever written or contributed to a newsgroup or, sometimes, mailing lists, is stored—for a short time anyway. It's all available for your searching, allowing for vast communicative and collaborative possibilities!

The search engines listed in this section are for finding information on the Internet's discussion forums (Usenet newsgroups) or on specific mailing lists. Many of the search engines reviewed earlier also allow searching within Usenet newsgroups.

I have also listed a few services that help you *find* mailing lists and news-groups. The software you use to read newsgroups also keeps a listing of all the current newsgroups. There is an advantage to using a subject guide in lieu of a search engine for simply finding a newsgroup or mailing list. These forums are typically more subject-specific, making it easier to locate an appropriate discussion. Such guides also generally offer a brief description of the newsgroup, whereas the software does not.

Most mailing lists' messages are not stored anywhere. This means you usually won't be able to find an archive of messages sent to that mailing list. This is actually quite a shame, because a lot of useful and meaningful discussion takes place in these forums—most of this is lost forever. For the few mailing lists that do keep archives, I will tell you how best to find those archives if they are on the Web. Some archives are found on the Web, while others can only be accessed through cryptic commands to the mailing list software. For the latter, the only sure method of finding out if an archive exists and how to access it is to contact the mailing list's owner. To help in this process, I have provided mailing lists owners' names and e-mail addresses in Chapter 6.

Resources below allow you to search for a specific subject found within a newsgroup, look for archives of mailing lists on the Web, find the name and address of a mailing list on a specific topic, or find a professional mailing list or newsgroup quickly.

Searching within Newsgroups

Title (or descriptor):	Google Groups
Owner:	Google
URL (Web address):	`http://groups.google.com/`
Rating:	★★★★

Google acquired the archive and technologies developed and refined by Deja.com, the pioneer in offering Web-based access to usenet, the Internet's discussion forums.

The advanced searching capabilities found in the original Deja are here, as well as a browseable directory of newsgroups and topics. As with Deja, the entire archive dating back to 1995 and comprising a terabyte of data, is available for searching. Newer posts to a newsgroup (within the most recent month) can also be replied to directly on the Web site.

Many people use a database of this nature to conduct research on people or what others' opinions are on a specific topic. For example, using Google Groups, you can view an author's entire posting history, including how many posts they made and to what specific groups. The advanced search form allows you to narrow your searches by newsgroup, author, message ID, language, or date.

Searching for Archives of Mailing Lists on the Web

You can utilize almost any search engine to look for an electronic mailing list or a mailing list's archives online, as long as you know the specific name of the list. This is not a foolproof method for finding mailing list archives, because the software that produces such archives is varied. Simply type the specific name of a mailing list into your favorite search engine. If the name is unique enough, the results will usually include information about the list and its archives online (if available). If the list's name is not unique, you can increase the likelihood of finding relevant results by typing in additional keywords related to the list's content. If these methods fail, your best bet is to use one of the search engines in the section below to find the list itself. Once found, the mailing list's general introductory file or Web site most often provides information about the list's archive and how to access it.

Searching for a Mailing List

Title (or descriptor):	Topica
Owner:	Topica, Inc
URL (Web address):	http://www.topica.com/
Rating:	★★★

With Topica's acquisition of Liszt, there is now no central, independent search engine for lists. Users are consigned to searching individual services, such as Topica and Yahoo! Groups. Topica is a mailing list hosting service that allows anyone to create and easily maintain a mailing list (and its archives) online at no cost. Hosting more than 100,000 lists currently, it's a much smaller and less feature-laden alternative to the enormous Yahoo! Groups (below).

Topica's search engine is a nightmare, returning only lists of categories initially. Some sample searches I conducted returned more than the first dozen or so pages of only categories, whereas individual mailing lists (the likely goal of most people's searches) follow. This is an unusual and user-hostile approach. Although Topica does provide results of mailing lists not hosted by its site (a la the old Liszt search), these come at the very end and are unlikely to be seen by anyone.

Title (or descriptor):	Yahoo! Groups
Owner:	Yahoo!, Inc.
URL (Web address):	http://groups.yahoo.com/
Rating:	★★★★

Yahoo! acquired and incorporated eGroups into its Web site, while retaining all of eGroups' outstanding functionality. Allowing anyone to start a new e-mail-based discussion group on any topic, Yahoo! Groups only requires registration for a free account. With more than 1 million groups available, this site is clearly the leader in online mail groups. One reason is the enhanced features it offers, which help to increase the interactivity of the group. These features include chat, file sharing, shared database access, polling, a calendar, and shared bookmarks. By using these features, members of a group can increase the cohesiveness and sense of community—two important aspects that can often be difficult to achieve online.

Searching for a Professional Mailing List or Newsgroup

Title (or descriptor):	Psych Central
Owner:	John M. Grohol, PsyD
URL (Web address):	http://psychcentral.com/
Rating:	★★★

In my humble opinion, Psych Central offers one of the better and more up-to-date listings of professional mailing lists and newsgroups in the areas of mental health, psychology, psychiatry, and social work. While not as comprehensive as Liszt, it is easier to use, allowing you to locate lists more quickly. Since the index is updated twice a month, it is also current and accurate. I would recommend checking out a guide like this first. Then, if you haven't found what you need, go wrestle search engines such as Goggle or Yahoo! for the information.

Getting Answers to Your Professional Questions

In this section of the book, I'll tell you how to find answers to commonly asked professional questions. Out of the hundreds of questions that have come to me via e-mail throughout the years, I've chosen some of the most interesting. Not only do I show you where to look online for these answers, but in most cases, I also tell you how I found this information in the first place. You can then conduct your own intelligent searches for information beyond that covered within this book.

3

Finding Disorders, Subspecialties, Clinical, and Treatment Information Online

This chapter helps you find basic information online about mental disorders, diagnosis, treatment, and subspecialty areas of professional interest. Such areas contain not only Web resources about alcoholism and substance abuse, neuropsychology, and trauma, but also social work, managed care, personality, and medication information.

As of this writing, there is no central Internet location for up-to-date, comprehensive treatment information; it is scattered throughout the online world. This is partly due to the multiple professions involved in the mental health field. While the lack of a central location may be disappointing at first, in truth it means that you can find a diversity of refereed opinions online from which to read and choose.

ARE DIAGNOSTIC CODES, CRITERIA, AND INFORMATION ONLINE FOR THE DSM-IV, ICD-9-CM, AND ICD-10?

It is very handy to have diagnostic categories, codes, and information on diagnoses available through online resources. Various Web sites, therefore, have made such information available at no cost to you. The *International Classification of Diseases* (ICD) is used widely except in the United States to diagnose and treat mental disorders. The latest version is the ICD-10, but the ICD-9-CM is still in common use. The *Diagnostic and Statistical Manual of Mental Disorders* (DSM) is utilized in the United States and elsewhere and is published by the American Psychiatric Association (APA). Through the "fair use" provision of U.S. copyright court decisions, parts of it have been made available online. The APA apparently has little intention of putting the entire manual online, though, because it is a primary income source for the association (much as PsycLIT and PsychINFO are income sources for the American Psychological Association). Understanding the economics behind organizations helps us understand why some reference material and databases are online when others are not.

Title (or descriptor):   Diagnostic Related Groups (DRGs)

Owner: Health Services Research Group

URL (Web address):

    `http://www.newcastle.edu.au/centre/hsrg/hypertexts/andrg.html`

Rating: ★★★

Need to look up a diagnostic related group code? This quick index of DRGs is one page long and very easy to use.

Title (or descriptor):   DSM-IV Diagnoses and Codes

Owner: Dr. Bob's Virtual En-psych-lopedia (Robert Hsiung, MD)

URL (Web address):   `http://www.dr-bob.org/tips/dsm4a.html`
    (Alphabetical listing)

URL (Web address):   `http://www.dr-bob.org/tips/dsm4n.html`
    (Ordered by diagnostic code)

Rating: ★★★

Straightforward presentation of the DSM-IV listing of mental disorders, either alphabetized by disorder or arranged by diagnostic code.

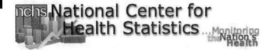

National Center for Health Statistics...Monitoring the Nation's Health

Title (or descriptor):	ICD-9-CM/ICD-10-M
Owner:	National Center for Health Statistics
URL (Web address):	http://www.cdc.gov/nchs/icd9.htm
Rating:	★★★★

Owner:	Health Services Research Group
URL (Web address):	

http://www.newcastle.edu.au/centre/hsrg/hypertexts/
icd9cm.html (Diagnostic codes only)

Rating:	★★

Owner:	American Hospital Association
URL (Web address):	http://www.ahacentraloffice.org/
Rating:	★★

Owner:	Yaki Technologies
URL (Web address):	http://www.eicd.com/
Rating:	★★★

Need an ICD-9-CM or ICD-10-CM code? The first site is the most comprehensive site of ICD-related information, including a bevy of word processing files that house the diagnostic codes, drug lists, and disease descriptions. The second site gives you easy online access to ICD-9-CM diagnostic codes. The Central Office Web site provides coding advice, workbooks, and information. The Yaki Technologies site provides a keyword- or code-searchable database of the ICD-9-CM online.

Title (or descriptor):	ICD-10 (Chapter V(F))
Owner:	Medical University of Lübeck, Department of Psychiatry & Fachhochschule Lübeck, Germany

URL (Web address):

`http://www.informatik.fh-luebeck.de/icd/welcome.html`

Owner: Internet Mental Health

URL (Web address):

`http://www.mentalhealth.com/` (by disorder)

Owner: World Health Organization

URL (Web address):   `http://www.who.int/whosis/icd10/`

Rating: ★★★

The first ICD-10 resource listed is a work-in-progress. When first visited, they had only completed the first two categories of the ICD-10's mental health section. Little progress had been noted in subsequent visits. Internet Mental Health hosts complete ICD-10 descriptions of 52 mental disorders on its site and is the best place to look for such information. The World Health Organization's site not only offers the complete categorical codes for the ICD-10's mental health section, but also ordering information for the ICD-10 itself.

HOW CAN I FIND UP-TO-DATE TREATMENT INFORMATION ONLINE?

There are places online where you can go to keep up with the latest interesting developments within the treatment field. There are two main types of resources: (1) those that directly provide you with treatment information through peer-reviewed research studies, articles, or news; and (2) those that can help you locate such research studies, articles, or news resources. Research articles and studies generally appear only in professionals journals, newspapers, or newsletters. Locating professional journals online to help track down treatment information, among many other uses, is described in Chapter 9.

Additional information resources include a number of online news services. News articles tend to be more watered-down and won't provide much useful content, but they may provide guidance on where to find additional information. Such news articles or press releases can also make you aware of development or government approval of new psychotropic medications. You can also use a search engine to find specific treatment information, using the steps outlined in Chapter 2.

Finding Clinical Information Directly on the Web

Title (or descriptor):   AmoebaWeb

Owner: Douglas Degelman, PhD

URL (Web address):

    `http://www.vanguard.edu/faculty/ddegelman/amoebaweb/`

Rating: ★★★

AmoebaWeb is a resource directory that not only provides professionals and students with information to clinical resources, but broader psychological resources as well. Simply designed with no advertising and few graphics, it is arranged in a logical, hierarchical format with categories such as applied, cognitive, developmental, marriage and family, school, social, and sport psychology. Broader psychological categories cover research methods, statistics, emotion and motivation, ethical issues, intelligence, language, and learning. It is regularly updated and has its own search engine that helps locate a specific resource fast. The biggest drawback is that none of the links are annotated, so you are never quite sure what you will find after clicking on one.

Title (or descriptor):   APApractice.org

Owner: APA Practice Organization

URL (Web address):   `http://www.apapractice.org/`

Rating: ★★★

This is a newer online service offered by the American Psychological Association's (APA) Practice Organization. It replaces the old, free PsycPractitioner Web site, which provided an information and news portal for clinicians. The new site is much larger and not as dependent as the old site was on the APA for its content. Its main categories include Legislative and Legal Advocacy, Practice Resources, Professional Development, Special Projects, Public Education Campaign, News and Publications, Products and Services, Books, Events, and more. Each section provides the kind of in-depth information that you would expect from a national organization. I hope to see more consistency in the amount and quality of information provided, however, as different sections had varying amounts of resources available. Some sections provided full-text articles (the default expectation), whereas others had only links to purchase a book on the topic. Overall the site provided a wealth of valuable information of relevance to its practitioner members.

AWARDS, BADGES, AND POPULARITY RATINGS ON THE WEB

"Popularity ratings" for various sites are featured on Internet Mental Health and on other places on the Web. Such ratings are one way Web sites try to distinguish themselves in a crowd. The myriad Web "badges" or "awards," handed out by dozens of different (and often competing) Web reviewers is an example of a similar phenomenon. Bestowing an "award badge" for a popular Web site goes back to the early days of the World Wide Web. One young upstart company called Point (now owned by Lycos) was looking for a way to make a name for itself online and ultimately become more marketable as a company. The Point "Top 5% of the Web" award badges were an instant success when they were first launched. They garnered Point the expected publicity and increased the volume of visitors to its own Web site. But this started an "award" phenomenon that has resulted in the creation of hundreds of award badges. The more awards given out, the less meaningful they—as a whole—become.

How strong a recommendation is such an award and how are they really chosen? Point relied on the badge's name ("Top 5% of the Web") to obtain its respectability, rather than a top-drawer editorial staff to do the actual reviews and ratings. The badge's claim of "Top 5%" should not be taken literally. It would be impossible to actually conduct such a rating service without in-depth statistical analyses of popularity, usability, quality, etc. They may just as well be the top 2%, the top 10%, or the top 30% of the Web. There's no actual way of measuring such a percentage. *Forbes Magazine,* among many other organizations, hands out "Best of the Web" awards online.

One way to determine a Web site's popularity is by counting the number of links that point to that site. The number of links to any given Web site, not including the site's own pages, can be estimated using the AltaVista and Google search engines. These derived "popularity ratings" are inaccurate and misleading for a number of reasons: (1) Search engines do not index all of the World Wide Web; it is not clear exactly how inclusive they really are. The amount of the Web indexed by each search engine also varies widely. (2) Some search engines, like AltaVista, are dynamic. This means that they are constantly changing (new entries are being added and deleted all the time), so the numbers returned will never be reliable. (3) Web sites themselves are dynamic and may change their Web addresses from time to time as they move (just like you change your home address from time to time). They may also offer different Web addresses that go to the same site. Popularity ratings are inaccurate and invalid if they don't address all of these concerns.

I suggest you forgo putting any serious weight into such ratings or award badges, as they have shown little differentiating value.

In order to gain access to this site, you have to be an APA member in good standing and pay the special assessment fee that is required of licensed psychologists. The APA's regular practice site, `http://www.apa.org/practice/`, also provides similar resources.

Title (or descriptor):	At Health Practitioner Connection
Owner:	At Health, Inc.
URL (Web address):	`http://www.athealth.com/Practitioner/`
Rating:	★★★★

Gradually developed over the past few years, At Health has emerged as a valuable resource to clinicians. Well-designed in a clean, thoughtful environment, At Health's Practitioner Connection provides access to timely and useful articles, a weekly newsletter, a medications database, professional tools, a bookstore, a professional directory tied to its consumer site, and a large offering of continuing education courses available for taking online. "Friday's Progress Notes" is a helpful professional newsletter published every other week on specific topics, such as practice management or substance abuse. Unlike other resources cluttered by advertisements or corporate imaging, At Health's focus on clinical content makes it a refreshing site to visit.

Title (or descriptor):	HelpHorizons Virtual Office
Owner:	HelpHorizons.com, Inc
URL (Web address):	`http://www.helphorizons.com/vo/`
Rating:	★★★

The HelpHorizons' Virtual Office offers a free library of professional articles and series that are targeted toward practicing mental health professionals. Although I'm an advisor for this company, the breadth and depth of content found in the articles speak for themselves. The "Steps to Success in Private Practice" is a very good series and, like all articles found in the library, is written in a down-to-earth style by a practitioner with direct tips and useful advice. The library is broken into four categories: clinical research updates, good business practices, billing tips, and online counseling, and it is completely searchable. With more than 100 articles online, the HelpHorizons Virtual Office is a valuable contribution to the online community.

Title (or descriptor):	Internet Mental Health
Owner:	Phillip W. Long, MD
URL (Web address):	`http://www.mentalhealth.com/`
Rating:	★★★

A general place to find treatment information is Internet Mental Health, which offers research citations and suggested bibliographies for many mental disorders. This Web site is a virtual encyclopedia of information related to mental disorders, their possible causes, and some treatments. It offers a relatively short list of links to other Web sites, organized by category and carrying "popularity ratings" (see box). Under certain disorders (the information available, such as diagnostic criteria, treatment guidelines, bibliographies, research abstracts, etc., varies greatly), readers will also find the ICD-10 criteria for the disorder, as well as Dr. Long's own diagnostic criteria for each. This latter section is of questionable value to most professionals, since we all conceptualize disorders quite differently. Furthermore, in the United States the DSM is the book used to diagnose mental disorders in most hospitals, institutions, and universities.

Internet Mental Health is vast, and is filled with tidbits from the "Harvard Mental Health Letter," "Medical Post," and other publications. It links to publications put out by the National Institute of Mental Health and others on disorders as well. It is one of the top mental health sites online today because of its cornucopia of knowledge on mental disorders. Readers will probably find some interesting and useful information on specific disorders nearly every time they visit the site.

Internet Mental Health is very much medically oriented and talks at great length about various medications and their use with some mental disorders. But be careful about taking the resource as a peer-reviewed and general mental health guide, because the information comes from a lone psychiatrist in Canada. While I didn't find anything overtly harmful in his general treatment guidelines, I did find his omission of social science research in general (which would not support some of his treatment recommendations) somewhat disturbing. The site itself is very large but lacks any search options. Its reliance on frames (dividing the Web browser's screen into smaller sections) to lay out information is unfortunate. For people who use small screens, this choice will make the Web site difficult to read and navigate. Its reliance on numerous but tiny graphics can also make the site slow to load.

Although Internet Mental Health continues to add new content to its site, the site's organization has become more confusing and cluttered with its antiquated frames-based layout. The frames also hide the fact that many links on the site actually point to other site's content. This type of questionable editorial linking while surrounding other sites' content with your own navigation is not only confusing to most users, but also potentially deceptive.

Title (or descriptor):	MDchoice.com
Owner:	MDchoice.com, Inc
URL (Web address):	`http://www.mdchoice.com/`
Rating:	★★★

MDchoice.com, Inc., which also owns the HealthScout news network, provides this valuable research tool. By entering as a professional, you will be able to search a large peer-reviewed database of reputable journal articles, presentations, practice guidelines, book chapters, videos, continuing education courses, and patient information resources. Although I don't care for the unfortunate layout of the site and its numerous advertisements, its search capabilities are a unique and valuable addition to the health world.

Using Guides to Find Additional Clinical Information Online

Unlike the two sites reviewed in the above section, the Web sites below simply link to other online resources that may provide additional clinical information on a wide range of subjects.

Title (or descriptor):	Behavioral Health World
Owner:	Essex Consulting, Inc.
URL (Web address):	`http://www.bhworld.com/`
Rating:	★★★

Behavioral Health World bills itself as a one-stop resource for substance abuse professionals, and it largely lives up to its mission. The site includes an extensive resource library, clinical case examples, a large continuing education event calendar, a research studies recruiting database, an online store for professionals, and a very inactive professional discussion forum. The large library of resources is divided into four major topic areas: client education, practitioner resources, research reports, and related resources. Each section contains public domain articles and links to additional sites of interest. The clinical case examples allow registered members (registration is free, but limited to qualified professionals only) to post cases of interest and receive other members' feedback on them. This well-designed site has potential for substance abuse (and more general mental health) professionals.

Title (or descriptor):   Medical Matrix–Psychiatry
Owner: Healthtel Corporation
URL (Web address):
    `http://www.medmatrix.org/_SPages/Psychiatry.asp`
Rating: ★★

Reviewed in-depth in Chapter 2, this site hosts a select list of psychiatric resources with brief descriptions.

Title (or descriptor):   MedWeb
Owner: Emory University Health Sciences Center Library
URL (Web address):   `http://www.medweb.emory.edu/MedWeb/`
Rating: ★★

MedWeb, from Emory University, is a medical directory that has been around for many years. During that time, it has undergone numerous revisions, but the most recent is by far the most usable. It still lacks the refinement found in more popular and well-known directories, but it is a step up from the numerous lists of links found elsewhere online. Links are categorized by topic areas, and brief descriptions are provided. A "What's New" section lets users know what has recently been added or updated in their database.

Title (or descriptor):	National Mental Health Information Center
Owner:	U.S. Department of Health and Human Services, Substance Abuse and Mental Health Services Administration, and the Center for Mental Health Services
URL (Web address):	http://www.mentalhealth.org/
Rating:	★★★★

An excellent U.S. government-sponsored Web site devoted to a wide range of mental health issues. The site includes links to mental health and substance abuse databases, a wealth of statistical data, as well as an extensive list of publications (many of which are available for downloading directly from the Web site, or may be ordered from the Web site).

Title (or descriptor):	Psych Central Psychology Resources
Owner:	John M. Grohol, PsyD
URL (Web address):	

http://psychcentral.com/resources/Psychology/

Rating:	★★★

This is my own regularly updated resource guide to professional resources online. The resource includes many additional subcategories, such as association and organization sites, managed care, continuing education, and journals and publications available online, and its database is searchable. Each resource listed includes a brief description and review, and is oriented toward mental health professionals looking for other helpful Web sites.

Title (or descriptor):	PsychScholar
Owner:	John Krantz, PhD
URL (Web address):	http://psych.hanover.edu/Krantz/
Rating:	★★★

This site hosts a great deal of psychology information. Included is a journal index, a listing of other psychology departments, an index to psychological societies, tutorials in psychology, links to software archives and other psychology-related sites. A good resource for college-level psychology courses.

Title (or descriptor):	Psych Web
Owner:	Russell A. Dewey, PhD
URL (Web address):	`http://www.psychwww.com/`
Rating:	★★★

Reviewed in-depth in Chapter 2. Extensive lists of links to other mental health and psychological resources make this a good place to start a search for treatment and clinical information.

Finding Treatment Information through a Search Engine

You can use a search engine (see also Chapter 2) to find references to articles or online documents that contain the actual treatment information. I'll use a simple example (treatment techniques for posttraumatic stress disorder) to guide us through this section. You may substitute nearly any disorder (e.g., depression, panic attacks, etc.) or treatment technique (EMDR, relaxation exercises, cognitive restructuring, hypnosis, NLP, etc.) to get similar results. Here's a couple of search terms I used in my search:

```
"treatment of PTSD"
"treatment of posttraumatic stress disorder"
"PTSD treatment"
"posttraumatic stress disorder treatment"
+PTSD +"new treatment"
```

You'll want to use quotation marks as noted, since these are specific phrases we're searching. (Note that there is no space between the plus sign and the quotation mark in the last example.) And since these are all different phrases, they will yield slightly different search results. You can probably think of a few others to try as well, if these don't provide you with the necessary information. Remember that you can always remove items from your search by using the negative sign (–) with most search engines. For example, if a herbal remedy kept appearing in your search results, simply append:

```
-herbal
```

to your search terms, and it will remove all results that contain the word "herbal." This also works for phrases enclosed in quotes as well as single words.

Using one of the methods discussed above, whether it be looking through journal listings, looking through the journals themselves from time to time, using search engines, or keeping track of health-related topics through news-oriented sites, you should be able to stay on top of the latest medical, health, and mental health developments in the treatment field. I would explore all of these options and find one that is reliable and works best for you. As with most things in life, there is no one "right" answer, only myriad competing but equally useful ones. Try them out and find the one right for you—the one that fits within your online habits and skills.

Keeping Up-to-Date with Online News Services

There are a few news services you can search and/or visit on a regular basis to keep abreast of the latest treatment developments. These news sites generally offer press releases and tidbits of information, which may or may not help the practicing clinician. If nothing else, they can keep the professional on top of the kind of "news" the general public is reading about mental health disorders and issues. This may be invaluable the next time a client walks into your office and asks, "So what do you think about that study announced yesterday that mental disorders are all biological?" You can become more prepared to answer such questions if you know the kinds of information that is being publicly disseminated. Reviewed below are the few that I recommend and visit regularly. "Access restrictions," found in some descriptions below, note any type of registration process and/or fee required before you can access the information found on that Web site.

Title (or descriptor):   CNN Health Section
Owner: CNN
URL (Web address):   http://www.cnn.com/HEALTH/
Rating: ★★★

The health section is updated daily with health and mental health-related stories.

Title (or descriptor):   Doctor's Guide–Psychiatric Disorders
Owner: Doctor's Guide Publishing Limited
URL (Web address):
   http://www.pslgroup.com/dg/psychiatrynews.htm
Rating: ★★

Doctor's Guide provides psychiatry news through a simple interface. The articles reside on the Doctor's Guide Web site but are often just republished press releases from pharmaceutical companies. It would be helpful if press releases were more clearly identified on the article index page, or even within the article itself. The site also provides updates from various psychiatry-related professional conferences. The psychiatry section is a part of the larger Doctor's Guide general medical news Web site.

Title (or descriptor):   Google News
Owner: Google
URL (Web address):   http://news.google.com/
Rating: ★★★★

Yes, Google does news, too. One of the more powerful and innovative areas that Google set its sights on back in 2002 was news headlines. Search engines have gotten pretty good at indexing regular Web content, but not always in the most timely of manners. Google News is a different kind of specialty search engine—it only indexes other news Web sites, but does so continuously. This means that if you are searching for the freshest news possible, on any topic, you should give Google News a try.

A simple query such as "depression treatment" (keep the quotation marks when typing in this query) led to dozens of stories published over the past few weeks. Some of them, such as news capsules published by television Web sites about a story they covered on a local news broadcast, are not very interesting. Others are press releases, published by a university or company promoting their recent research or drug study findings. Nevertheless, more often than not, this is the same information on which reporters base their stories. Rather than hearing the news filtered through a third-party reporter, you can keep updated on your research or clinical interests directly through Google News. It also is a great general news Web site, on any other subject category or topic that interests you, because it combines all the major news sources into one easy-to-use site.

Title (or descriptor):	HealthScout
Owner:	MDChoice.com, Inc.
URL (Web address):	`http://www.healthscout.com/`
Rating:	★★★

Although they do not have a specific mental health news category, this site is better known for providing health news to dozens of other sites via its syndication network. The site publishes original content by its own reporters, an unexpected feature that has become increasingly rare in the online world. Another unique feature of the site is that sources are directly noted within the original articles—no more need for a reader to guess how or where the reporter obtained his or her information. Updated daily, HealthScout also offers access to mainstream media articles on health.

Title (or descriptor):	Medscape
Owner:	WebMD, Inc.
URL (Web address):	`http://www.medscape.com/`
URL (Web address):	
	`http://www.medscape.com/edchoicedirectory/psychiatry`
Rating:	★★★
Access restrictions:	Registration required, free

Medscape, as its name implies, is oriented toward physicians and medical topics, but it carries a fair amount of information relevant to the field of psychology and mental health in its "Psychiatry" section.

Title (or descriptor):	News Is Free
Owner:	Mike Krus
URL (Web address):	http://www.newsisfree.com/
Rating:	★★★

Using this free headline aggregator, you can easily type in any keywords or phrases and find the latest news headlines from thousands of Web sites. Try keywords such as "mental health," "psychology," or "psychiatry" to get you started. Beware, though. News Is Free doesn't differentiate between respected, reliable news Web sites and Web logs (or "blogs," individuals' online personal journals). Blogs are often filled with personal opinion, insights, and unrelated material that may have little to do with your query. However, if you are looking for something a little different in your news online, this is a great site to visit.

Title (or descriptor):	Open Minds
Owner:	Open Minds
URL (Web address):	http://www.openminds.com/
Rating:	★★★
Access restrictions:	Free and subscription sections

Open Minds is a behavioral health care consulting firm that offers updated industry news free on their site. For a fee, they offer access to their informative newsletters on-line, including their namesake newsletter, Open Minds. Open Minds also provides access to industry and government reports, white papers, and publications. For administrators and managers in behavioral health care, a subscription to Open Minds is usually a necessary part of doing business.

Title (or descriptor):	PsychLinx
Owner:	MDLinx, Inc.
URL (Web address):	http://www.mdlinx.com/psychlinx/index.cfm
Rating:	★★

A specialty news Web site for psychiatry professionals, PsychLinx provides abstracts from recent journal articles and select news stories from general news sources. It is a subsection of the larger, medically oriented MDLinx, and a free registration is required to access the articles. The article links lead to the article's actual location on various external Web sites, which can be a bit tedious to navigate. Sometimes the links simply led to a journal's home page, and I had to navigate further on my own to find the actual article. The summaries are not dated, so you don't know how recent they are until you click through to the article.

Title (or descriptor):	Reuters Health
Owner:	Reuters, Inc.
URL (Web address):	`http://www.reutershealth.com/`
Rating:	★★★
Access restrictions:	Registration required; free and subscriptions sections

Although mainly oriented toward general health and medical topics, Reuters often publishes relevant and useful clinical information on mental disorders. News briefs are updated daily. Reuters Medical News, a subsection of the site oriented toward healthcare professionals, is available for an annual subscription.

Title (or descriptor):	USA Today
Owner:	USA Today
URL (Web address):	

`http://www.usatoday.com/news/healthscience/hsfront.htm`

Rating:	★★★

This Web site includes daily news, as well as in-depth reports, such as *USA Today*'s objective look at the use of electroconvulsive therapy (ECT) as a treatment for depression.

WHERE CAN I FIND CLINICAL INFORMATION ONLINE IN SUBSPECIALTY AREAS?

Hundreds of professionals maintain Web sites devoted to specific professional topics, ranging from alcohol resources and neuropsychology, to managed care and dealing with childhood trauma. Many other Web sites are maintained by government or academic organizations. The authors of these sites have put considerable resources and effort into providing not just information about their particular organization or interests, but also about a wide range of clinical and research topics. Most of these sites are of high quality (or I wouldn't bother listing them here) and are relatively stable. This means you can visit them and will probably find useful information, pointers to additional resources in that topic area (both online and in the real world), and you can trust that the information is reasonably accurate.

Most of the resources for specific areas listed next in this chapter have been gathered from the various large indexes (found in Chapter 2 and earlier in this chapter). You may use such indexes, search engines, and search guides to find other specific sites on areas covered below or other topics of interest. The balance of this chapter is just a small sampling of the hundreds of useful and valuable Web sites maintained by professionals for professionals.

Adler, Freud, Jung, and Psychoanalysis Online

Title (or descriptor):   Classical Adlerian Psychology

Owner: Henry T. Stein, PhD

URL (Web address):

    `http://ourworld.compuserve.com/homepages/hstein/`

Rating: ★★★

One of the oldest sites on the Web for Adlerian psychology, this site includes dozens of articles on theory, philosophy, theology, and practice. It offers biographical information on Adler and others in a simple but well-designed site, which is updated frequently. The site also features a companion discussion forum on Behavior Online.

Title (or descriptor):   C. G. Jung Home Page

Owner: Donald Williams, LPC

URL (Web address):   `http://www.cgjungpage.org/`

Rating: ★★★

Everything about Jung, including a glossary of Jungian terms, abstracts, articles, and links to many other analytic and Jungian resources. This site is constantly updated and well maintained.

Title (or descriptor):	New York Psychoanalytic Institute
Owner:	New York Psychoanalytic Institute
URL (Web address):	`http://psychoanalysis.org/`
Rating:	★★★

This resource-rich site of the New York Psychoanalytic Institute offers a great deal of knowledge and information about Sigmund Freud and psychoanalysis. In addition to the Institute's own articles, the site provides links to other Freud resources online, educational and training courses, treatment and referral information, meetings and events, and funding opportunities.

Title (or descriptor):	Psychoanalysis–Techniques and Practice
Owner:	Romanian Association for Psychoanalytic Promotion
URL (Web address):	

`http://www.freudfile.org/psychoanalysis/`

Rating:	★★★

A site discussing themes and techniques of psychoanalysis.

Alcoholism and Substance Abuse Online

Title (or descriptor):	Alcoholism/Substance Abuse
Owner:	About, Inc.
URL (Web address):	`http://alcoholism.about.com/`
Rating:	★★★

The Alcoholism/Substance Abuse site, part of the About.com network, is a wonderful, constantly updated resource. It offers information about all the basics, including Alcoholics Anonymous and 12-step programs in general. The site's guide is a recovering alcoholic, not a professional, so the resources chosen and highlighted may sometimes reflect that person's experiences and preferences. The hundreds of About.com sites all act as large-scale resources for their individual topics, maintained by volunteer experts who get paid based upon the popularity of their About.com site. Unfortunately, this results in a wealth of annoying pop-up and pop-under advertisements filling your computer screen, detracting from the content of the sites themselves.

Title (or descriptor):	Dual Diagnosis Website
Owner:	Kathleen Sciacca
URL (Web address):	http://www.erols.com/ksciacca/
Rating:	★★

With over a half-dozen articles about the treatment of dually diagnosed patients (substance or alcohol abuse with an existing mental disorder), a bibliography, links to other online resources, a discussion forum, and an interactive chat area, this is a well-designed, informative site.

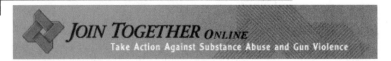

Title (or descriptor):	Join Together
Owner:	Join Together
URL (Web address):	http://www.jointogether.org/
Rating:	★★★★

One of the premier sites online today for alcohol, substance abuse, and gun violence information, legislative alerts, resources, news, and updates. A well-designed and attractive site makes finding information (including news headlines, grants, and community organizations) on alcohol, substance abuse, and drug violence easy.

Title (or descriptor):	PrevLine: National Clearinghouse for Alcohol and Drug Information
Owner:	Center for Substance Abuse Prevention, Substance Abuse and Mental Health Services Administration, and Center for Substance Abuse Treatment
URL (Web address):	http://www.health.org/
Rating:	★★★★

In a crowded field of excellent substance abuse resources online directed toward professionals, PrevLine still manages to stand out. Includes fact sheets, research news and updates, and a wealth of online resource guides. A powerful search engine makes any topic easy to find, and the pleasant, consistent look of the site makes it easy to navigate.

Title (or descriptor):	Substance Abuse and Mental Health Services Administration
Owner:	Substance Abuse and Mental Health Services Administration (SAMHSA)
URL (Web address):	http://www.samhsa.gov/
Rating:	★★★★

This site provides a starting point to jump to a number of important government resources related to not only substance abuse but mental health in general, including the Center for Mental Health Services (CMHS), the Center for Substance Abuse Prevention (CSAP), the Center for Substance Abuse Treatment, the National Clearinghouse for Alcohol and Drug Information (PrevLine, above), and the National Mental Health Services Knowledge Exchange Network (KEN). Reports, data, statistical information, grants, and further resources may be found at each of these sites.

Title (or descriptor):	Web of Addictions
Owner:	Andrew L. Homer, PhD, and Dick Dillon
URL (Web address):	http://www.well.com/user/woa/
Rating:	★★

A large, comprehensive site where information on drug and addiction topics is easily found. A global listing of fact sheets on addictions residing on over a dozen different Web servers around the world is especially invaluable. A meeting and conference calendar and links to other addiction resources online, such as Alcoholics Anonymous and lots of recovery-oriented sites, are also available. Unfortunately, the site has suffered in recent years from few updates, resulting in many links that no longer work.

Assessment and Testing

Title	Performance Assessment Network (PAN)
Owner:	Performance Assessment Network
URL:	http://www.pantesting.com/
Rating:	★★★★

The Performance Assessment Network (PAN) brings together under one umbrella Web site hundreds of assessment instruments from dozens of test publishers. A growing number of these measures are available online, directly through the PAN Web site. What that means is a simplification and standardization of the testing process. For example, a client can be directed by their clinician to log onto the site to take a specific test or a customized battery of tests. The clinician then logs on and finds that the test has been automatically scored, complete with a report (in an area called the "PAN box"). All the data and logins are protected by the Web's security protocol, SSL, an encryption technology built in to everybody's Web browser. It is apparent that a great deal of thought and effort went into designing the online test-taking experience through the site.

Tests are available in a dozen major categories, such as Personality and Personal Skills Assessment, Pre-Employment Screening, Self-Development, Clinical Assessment Tools, IT Skills, and Organizational Surveys, among others. Clicking on a test name within a category results in a more detailed description, including what the test measures, the publisher, and the user level needed to access it. What is missing, however, is the cost of using the test (which is available to registered members). Test manuals and sample reports are also available to properly authorized and registered users for any test they wish to administer. While many of the measures available on the site are not commonly recognized, most do have validated psychometrics.

PAN is sensitive to the protected nature of many psychological instruments and allows only qualified professionals varying access levels to protected tests. The site categorizes the level of test protection according to a simple four-stage system. Level A tests offer the highest protection and are available only to licensed clinicians at the doctoral level. Level B tests are available to graduate-level educated professionals. Both levels A and B are generally reserved for clinical and personality measures. Level C tests, the most common level of tests found on the site, only require a bachelor's level education in psychology (or related fields) and demonstrated experience in use of assessments. Level D tests are noncontrolled, meaning that anyone can access them.

Title (or descriptor):	PsychTests
Owner:	Plumeus, Inc.
URL (Web address):	`http://www.psychtests.com/`
Rating:	★★★

Unlike the Performance Assessment Network (PAN, above), PsychTests offers a strictly independent approach to psychological online testing. PsychTests assessments are created in-house, validated, and published exclusively through one of their Web sites (Queendom.com is the public version of the site). Similar to PAN, however, PsychTests offers a customized area where professionals log in and view the test results of their clients (called the ARCH Profile system). Consumers can also log in to their own profile section, which allows them to keep track of their test results over time. A smaller selection of tests is available, but their pricing model is much less expensive as well (a flat fee of $12.75/month at the time of this writing, with volume discounts available). With no per-use fees, this model is very attractive to clinicians on a budget.

There are presently over five dozen tests on the site, categorized within five major topic areas: intelligence, relationship and love, personality, career, and health. The tests range from 32-item assertiveness and 40-item procrastination tests, to 85-item depression and 30-item anxiety quizzes. Unlike PAN, PsychTests' site displays banner advertising, a distracting element on the top of each page, but likely this helps to keep costs lower. PsychTests provides an independent, legitimate, and useful alternative to a site like PAN and is recommended for the independent practitioner.

Clinicians' Directories

There are a lot of Web sites that provide directories of mental health professionals online (see `http://dmoz.org/Health/Mental_Health/Counseling_Services/Directories/` for a general listing), but I'm just going to draw your attention to two below that appear to stand out above the crowd. For cheap, easy marketing online, clinicians should consider registering with as many free online directories as possible, but they need to consider more carefully those services requiring an annual fee.

Title (or descriptor):	Find-a-Therapist.com
Owner:	Find-a-Therapist.com, Inc.
URL (Web address):	`http://www.find-a-therapist.com/`
Rating:	★★★

A solid, well-designed offering, Find-a-Therapist.com provides consumers a place to go to quickly find a clinician within their local community. Acting as a virtual Yellow Pages, this specialized directory costs nothing for therapists to add their basic listing to it, but more detailed listings begin at $50 annually and go as high as $245 annually. Find-a-Therapist also offers a smaller e-therapy directory of providers. Overall, the site appears to be an emerging service worthy of consideration.

Title (or descriptor):	Search for Therapists and Treatment Facilities
Owner:	CenterSite, LLC
URL (Web address):	

`http://mentalhelp.net/poc/view_index.php/idx/14`

Rating:	★★★

One of the older databases online, the Mental Help Net therapist directory benefits from a strong consumer mental health site built around it, driving hundreds of potential referrals to the service every day. A listing for therapy within the database is free, with virtually no limit to the amount of personal and professional information you can add to your entry, so it makes sense to put your practice in it. Like other directory services, once registered, users can readily update their listings to reflect changes in their practice. Enhanced listings are available for a $120 annual fee.

Title (or descriptor):	Therapist Directory
Owner:	Psychology.com, Inc.
URL (Web address):	`http://www.psychology.com/therapist/`
Rating:	★★

The greatest benefit in registering with this directory service for $100 annually is its old, sought-after domain name. Lots of people visit Psychology.com because it is the default site you get to when you type in the word "psychology" into most Web browsers' Address field.

Forensic Psychiatry and the Law Online

Title (or descriptor):	Psychiatry & the Law
Owner:	James F. Hooper, MD, University of Alabama and the Alabama Department of Mental Health and Mental Retardation

URL (Web address):

    `http://bama.ua.edu/~jhooper/tableofc.html`

Rating: ★★★

A very large and well-maintained resource of law decisions related to mental health, psychiatry, and psychology. The link labeled "Landmark cases in mental health law" provides useful plain-English case summaries of U.S. court cases that directly affect mental health practice.

Managed Care Online

Title (or descriptor):	Open Minds
Owner:	Open Minds
URL (Web address):	`http://www.openminds.com/`
Rating:	★★★

Open Minds is a research and consulting firm that's as well known in the behavioral health care industry as KPMG is to the financial services world. Their Web site has grown over the years and now offers an emerging set of resources that are of value to administrators and clinicians trying to make sense of the industry. In addition to their popular print newsletters (online access is available to their articles for subscribers), Open Minds offers information about upcoming workshops and seminars, publications, and other resources that try to make sense of managed care.

Title (or descriptor):	Policy Information Exchange (PIE) Online
Owner:	Missouri Institute of Mental Health (MIMH)
URL (Web address):	`http://www.mimh.edu/mimhweb/pie/`
Rating:	★★★

This service acts as a central clearinghouse for mental health and behavioral health-care policy data, information, legislative and policy updates, and press and news releases. Links and news are regularly updated, and include updates of legislative developments on both the federal and state levels. A searchable calendar of related conferences and events is available, as is a literature search service (for a fee) through the MIMH library. PIE Online's main database is fully searchable, and the site is easy to navigate. The site unfortunately lacks information about PIE's purpose and history.

Title (or descriptor):	Psychotherapy Finances Online
Owner:	Psychotherapy Finances
URL (Web address):	`http://www.psyfin.com/`
Rating:	★★★

Although largely designed to help sell new subscriptions to their publication *Psychotherapy Finances*, this site provides numerous news updates every month from each of these newsletters. The publisher also offers weekly-updated news links, the table of contents of each newsletter online, and hosts a discussion forum and provider directory on the site. This is a growing site which provides some good business resources for behavioral health providers.

Medications and Psychopharmacology References Online

Title (or descriptor):	*The Merck Manual of Diagnosis and Therapy*
Owner:	Merck & Co, Inc.
URL (Web address):	`http://www.merck.com/`
Rating:	★★★

Sections of the venerable Merck Manual are available for free reading online. While not specifically a psychopharmacology book, it does offer some treatment guidelines and recommendations for all the major mental disorders. It is also a good overall psychiatric resource for mental health professionals to understand more about mental disorders in general.

Title (or descriptor):	Psychopharmacology Tips
Owner:	Robert Hsiung, MD
URL (Web address):	`http://www.dr-bob.org/tips/`
Rating:	★★

An older archive of drug knowledge for professionals looking for some of the lore about how best to prescribe psychotropic medications. Arranged according to types of medications, as well as problem areas, this site is relatively easy to use. Information found here is no longer updated and so should be used with caution. The tips were originally drawn by Dr. Hsiung from the psychopharmacology professional mailing list.

Title (or descriptor):	RxList
Owner:	RxList, LLC
URL (Web address):	http://www.rxlist.com/
Rating:	★★★★

A complete reference of over 4,000 drugs available for searching. The results give only the brand name, generic name, and class of drug. The "Top 200 Prescriptions" are available with generic prescribing information. Professional and growing, this is usually a reliable and stable source of basic medication information.

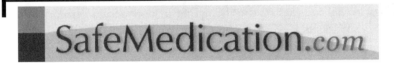

Title (or descriptor):	SafeMedication.com
Owner:	American Society of Health-System Pharmacists
URL (Web address):	http://www.safemedication.com/
Rating:	★★★★

A simple, easy-to-use online drug database is difficult to find. Many sites clutter their pages with advertisements or make you browse through hundreds of drug names in order to find the one you want. SafeMedication.com, published by the American Society of Healthy-System Pharmacists, is one of the best drug databases online today, because it offers a clean design with minimal graphics and no advertisements. You simply type in the drug's generic or brand name and it will display drugs that match that name. It even accepts misspellings, in case you are not sure exactly how to spell the medication you're searching for. Medication listings are written in plain English and tell you why a medication is prescribed, how it should be used, any special precautions, what to do when you forget a dose, side effects, storage and miscellaneous information. Although not as detailed or up to date with the latest medications as some other drug databases online, SafeMedication.com is a good standard site for professionals and their clients.

Title (or descriptor):	WebMD Health: Drugs & Herbs
Owner:	WebMD, Inc.
URL (Web address):	

```
http://my.webmd.com/medical_information/drug_and_herb/
drugs/
```

| Rating: | ★★★ |

As with any large health site online, WebMD offers access to a comprehensive drug database through its site. Although somewhat difficult to find and offering only a browseable list of medications (both generic and brand names are indexed), the site is comprehensive and thorough. It includes newer medications earlier than other online drug databases. Drug summaries are written in plain English, making them simple to understand. If you are tempted to type in a drug's name in WebMD's search engine, don't bother. For popular medications, the results will net you dozens of listings, even if you click on the "Drug Information" results category in an effort to narrow your search. It will be easier for most people to browse through the alphabetical Drugs & Herbs list provided here.

Neurophysiology, Neuropsychology, Neuroscience, and Biofeedback Online

Title (or descriptor):	Association for Applied Psychophysiology and Biofeedback
Owner:	Association for Applied Psychophysiology and Biofeedback
URL (Web address):	`http://www.aapb.org/`
Rating:	★★★

General information can be found on this Web site on biofeedback, clinical psychophysiology, and links to related resources online.

Title (or descriptor):	Books and Articles on the Brain & Neurophysiology
Owner:	William H. Calvin
URL (Web address):	`http://www.WilliamCalvin.com/`
Rating:	★★★

A large home page (which will take most computers a long time to load) offers a confusing array of choices. But many of the books William Calvin has written over the years on the brain, evolution, and future directions may be found here. Not just to purchase, mind you, but to read the full text of these books online.

Title (or descriptor):	Neuropsychology Central
Owner:	Jeff Browndyke
URL (Web address):	`http://www.neuropsychologycentral.com/`
Rating:	★★

A site largely made up of links to a great deal of neuropsychology resources online. The site's content is often eclipsed by its design, however, especially with its large home page graphics (which will take most computers a long time to load). Categories include assessment, geriatric, forensic, neuroimaging, treatment, and cognitive resources, among many others. Online discussion forums are also provided.

 Neurosciences on the Internet
<Neuroguide.com>

Title (or descriptor):	Neurosciences on the Internet
Owner:	Neil A. Busis, MD
URL (Web address):	`http://www.neuroguide.com/`
Rating:	★★★★

Offering a searchable database as well as extensive resources about the neurosciences, neuropsychology, and neuropsychiatry. The resources are well categorized and easy to find, and an internal search engine is included. The site is updated regularly with new resources and links to valuable information. Three international mirror sites are also available.

Personality Online

Title (or descriptor):	Great Ideas in Personality
Owner:	G. Scott Acton
URL (Web address):	http://www.personalityresearch.org/
Rating:	★★★★

This site acts as a great resource for general personality information as well as a dozen different personality theories. It includes original papers published on the site, a bibliography, a useful database of personality researchers around the world, an FAQ, glossary, and more. Professional resources include grants concerning personality, courses offered around the world in personality theory, and journals, societies and personality textbooks. Each subsection on different personality theories is a virtual mini-site, offering a wide breadth of information, resources, and suggested related readings. The whole site is simply designed making navigation and reading easy and pleasurable.

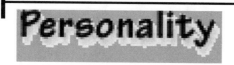

Title (or descriptor):	Personality and Consciousness
Owner:	Eric Pettifor
URL (Web address):	http://www.wynja.com/personality/
Rating:	★★★★

An excellent site devoted to discussing the major theorists in personality psychology, including Alfred Adler, Arnold Bruhn, Sigmund Freud, Carl Jung, George Kelly, Abraham Maslow, Carl Rogers, B. F. Skinner, and Charles T. Tart. The Web site offers not only their respective theories and philosophies on psychotherapy, but recommends related and worthwhile books.

Title (or descriptor):	The Personality Project
Owner:	William Revelle
URL (Web address):	http://www.personality-project.org/
Rating:	★★★

Although not as regularly updated as I would prefer, the Personality Project offers a great resource filled with a wealth of information relating to personality theory. The site covers personality taxonomies, assessment, applications, and theory. It neatly categorizes additional Internet resources into academic, nonacademic, and psychological organizations. The site features a section entitled, "Special advice for students," that provides additional articles and resources for students interested in studying personality and going to graduate school.

Posttraumatic Stress Disorder and Trauma Resources Online

Title (or descriptor):	National Center for PTSD
Owner:	National Center for PTSD, U.S. Department of Veterans Affairs
URL (Web address):	`http://www.ncptsd.org/`
Rating:	★★★★

A simple but accessible site for clinical and research information on posttraumatic stress disorder (PTSD). The PILOTS database ("Published International Literature on Traumatic Stress") is also maintained here. This database includes over 22,000 article titles and abstracts on trauma-related literature. National Center Fact Sheets offer information on selected aspects of PTSD, mainly for laypeople.

The site continues to grow and now offers a well-written FAQ and a Special Topics in PTSD section that covers recent wars, active duty information, anniversary reactions, and much more. Most popular pages are also highlighted so that you can quickly discover what is of interest to other visitors to the site.

Title (or descriptor):	Trauma Information Pages
Owner:	David Baldwin, PhD
URL (Web address):	`http://www.trauma-pages.com/`
Rating:	★★★★

Updated regularly, this site focuses primarily on emotional trauma and traumatic stress, including PTSD. Details not only possible causes and treatments of trauma, but also includes extensive lists of additional online resources in the trauma field. The academic articles on the site are primarily research articles on PTSD. The site has maintained a clean, simple design making it easy to navigate and read.

Title (or descriptor):   Trauma Treatment Manual
Owner: Ed Schmookler, PhD
URL (Web address):
    `http://www.amsterdam.park.org/Guests/Stream/`
    `trauma_manual.htm`
Rating: ★★

An online treatment manual that gives professionals an overview of trauma treatment from one psychologist's viewpoint. Includes treatment guidelines and examples.

Psychology and Religion Online

Title (or descriptor):   Psychology of Religion Pages
Owner: Michael Neilsen, PhD
URL (Web address):   `http://www.psychwww.com/psyrelig/`
Rating: ★★★

Offering original articles, essays, book reviews, and related resources online, this site provides a wealth of content about religion from a psychological point of view. Articles are in simple, plain text making reading them on this site a pleasure. Science and religious news updates are also provided.

School Psychology and Teaching Resources Online

Title (or descriptor):   School Psychology Resources Online
Owner: Sandy Steingart
URL (Web address):   `http://www.schoolpsychology.net/`
Rating: ★★★

An excellent compendium of resources for school psychology, including resource lists of common disorders and problems studied in this field.

Title (or descriptor):	Teaching Clinical Psychology
Owner:	John Suler
URL (Web address):	http://www.rider.edu/suler/tcp.html
Rating:	★★★

A great deal of information may be found on this well-constructed site about teaching clinical psychology, including in-class exercises, projects, suggested course syllabi, and reading materials. Essays and links to other related resources round out this site.

Social Work and Social Psychology Resources Online

Title (or descriptor):	Clinical Social Work Homepage
Owner:	Pat McClendon, MSSW, CSW
URL (Web address):	http://www.ClinicalSocialWork.com/
Rating:	★★

Articles of interest to social workers and assorted mental health resources, all of which are updated irregularly, make this a good page to visit.

Title (or descriptor):	Social Psychology Network
Owner:	Scott Plous, PhD
URL (Web address):	http://www.socialpsychology.org/
Rating:	★★★★

The Social Psychology Network has been a labor of love for Scott Plous of Wesleyan University since 1996. Growing from an original index of just a few dozen resources, the site now indexes thousands of social psychology and general psychology resources online. It includes a wealth of interesting resources, such as a ranking of psychology Ph.D. programs in the United States from a 1995 study; a software database; an excellent, comprehensive distance learning guide; and much more. Other sites within the Social Psychology Network are interesting diversions in themselves, such as JoeChemo.org (a parody of Joe Camel) and UnderstandingPrejudice.org. The site comes integrated with a powerful search engine and is regularly updated and maintained.

Title (or descriptor):	Social Work Access Network (SWAN)
Owner:	College of Social Work at the University of South Carolina
URL (Web address):	`http://www.sc.edu/swan/`
Rating:	★★★

An excellent resource for social workers, offering resources and links to associations and additional, general social work information. It appears to be irregularly updated these days.

Title (or descriptor):	Social Work World
Owner:	Liz Mitchell, MSW, LCSW, CISW
URL (Web address):	`http://socialworkworld.org/`
Rating:	★★

Social Work World is a simple site that offers interested readers information about social work through articles, updated news provided from Google News, and links to other social work resources around the world. The site also supports an active Yahoo! e-mail group of the same name and provides subscription instructions for it.

Statistical Help Online

Title (or descriptor):	SurfStat Australia
Owner:	Department of Statistics, The University of Newcastle–Australia
URL (Web address):	

`http://www.anu.edu.au/nceph/surfstat/surfstat-home/ surfstat.html`

Rating:	★★★★

SurfStat is a very nicely constructed general statistics resource and tutorial, providing all the basics of statistical analysis. Both framed and unframed versions are available from the above URL. Practice exercises and links to other statistical online resources are also available. A great online starting point for statistical information.

4

Locating Employment Opportunities through the Web

At one time or another, most of us seek new employment opportunities. It may be because we're moving for family reasons, or just looking for a change of pace, or we've been "downsized" out of a job. Going online is an excellent place to begin your search for a new job. There are dozens of large and useful employment databases online today, as well as a few hidden gems, which are a bit more difficult to find.

As with treatment information, there is no central online clearinghouse that lists all the available jobs for all mental health–related professions. You will, therefore, have to do some jumping around and visit a number of Web sites to ensure a thorough search. This situation is unlikely to change in the near future because of the vast variety of competing interests in listing employment opportunities, as well as the great number of differences among professions, which keeps such listings as scattered in the real world.

HOW DO I FIND JOB OPPORTUNITIES IN MENTAL HEALTH ONLINE?

Begin your search with an employment guide; a human-compiled collection of employment-related Web sites. Employment guides contain listings of databases for various online employment classified ads. Then select and visit the most relevant databases to see the actual employment ads themselves. I recommend two broad job guides to get you started; one specific to the mental health field and the other more general. Alternatively, you could go directly to one of the employment and career databases that I also list. It was through the employment guides that I discovered these services. This list is by no means comprehensive. I have, however, tried to choose from among the oldest, largest, and most interesting sites available.

Searching the Employment Guides

Title (or descriptor):	Open Directoy Project: Business: Employment
Owner:	Netscape
URL (Web address):	`http://www.dmoz.org/Business/Employment/`
Rating:	★★★

A smaller, less comprehensive listing than Yahoo's (below), the Open Directory Project provides another list of employment guides that may be of help.

Title (or descriptor):	Yahoo! Business and Economy: Employment: Jobs
Owner:	Yahoo!, Inc.
URL (Web address):	

`http://www.yahoo.com/Business_and_Economy/`
`Employment_and_Work/`

Rating:	★★★★

Yahoo! is known for its quality listings of online resources in myriad categories. Their resource lists are updated regularly by their large editorial staff, and their simple rating system ("cool" versus "not cool") may help you decide where to begin your search. This listing of employment databases is much larger than Mental Health Net's, but it includes many that will be of no relevance to mental health professionals. As with anything found on Yahoo!, there are one-line descriptions next to most resources, and the site itself is very well organized and usually quick to load (if not overly busy, as it often is in the later afternoon and evening hours).

Reading the Classified Ads Online: Employment and Career Databases

There are a lot of other, smaller, and more difficult-to-find databases of various employment opportunities also online. While you might find them with a search engine, the best way is to use one of the above guides as a starting point. I've listed below a few I found from the guides that are likely to be the most relevant to you.

Title (or descriptor):	America's Job Bank
Owner:	United States Department of Labor and local state public Employment Service Agencies
URL (Web address):	http://www.jobsearch.org/
Rating:	★★★★

This classified ad service is nationwide and allows you to search under any profession. My searches for "psychologist" and "mental" (as in "mental health professional" or "mental health counselor" or the like) both turned up over dozens of listings. This Web site is easy to use with appropriate graphics and a logical layout. It is one of the better large, nonspecific job sites. Information is presented in a familiar, standard format that includes the job title, location, salary, education and experience required, hours, and schedule (e.g., full time). As with all of the larger nationwide databases, America's Job Bank also allows searching by individual state, profession, and offers a self-directed occupational search. Using the latter method, I chose the "counseling" category and discovered over 250 jobs nationwide! One of the most useful government-sponsored sites on the Web today.

Title (or descriptor):   American Psychological Society Job Listings

Owner: American Psychological Society

URL (Web address):

    `http://www.psychologicalscience.org/jobs/`

Rating: ★★

From the American Psychological Society's *Observer,* the classified ads were search-able only by keyword when I visited the site. The keyword search makes it difficult to limit search results to certain geographical locations. You can, however, view the entire month's listings and use your Web browser's internal search function to find relevant jobs more easily.

Title (or descriptor):   CareerBuilder

Owner: CareerBuilder, Inc.

URL (Web address):   `http://www.careerbuilder.com/`

Rating: ★★★

CareerBuilder takes a slightly different approach to offering classified employment announcements. More than three dozen newspapers and 30 additional large sites such as MSN.com and Bloomberg.com have teamed up with CareerBuilder to offer employment classified ads in one, easy-to-use search engine. You can find ads rele-vant to your needs by choosing which of these sites you'd like to search, choosing a general job description (such as "Health & Medical"), then listing any additional key-words you'd like to use to further limit your search. The benefit of this approach is that you can easily search all of these databases without having to go to their individ-ual Web sites. This can also be a boon to those looking to relocate to a specific geo-graphical location. Twenty-five results are returned at a time, along with the title of the job, a brief description, and the job's geographical location. Overall, the site's user interface is simple to use, and the site is quick and responsive, an improvement from the site's previous incarnation.

Title (or descriptor):   Career Network

Owner: The Chronicle of Higher Education

URL (Web address):   `http://chronicle.com/jobs/`

Rating:	★★★
Access restrictions:	Optional registration

One of the more comprehensive job databases for the academic world, it offers a variety of flexible search methods to allow you to find relevant employment opportunities quickly and easily. It allows readers to either browse through listings, or search via keywords, and it offers one of the largest listings of positions available today. The version available to unregistered readers (registration is optional) is a compilation of employment listings that are 1 week old, but the most current version of the database is open to current subscribers to *The Chronicle of Higher Education*. Since this Web site is updated weekly and academic positions tend to be advertised for months, even the week-old listings are timely and probably current enough for most readers. Browsing through the job listings keeps you on their Web site, where the graphics are clean and the site is fast. If you're seeking an academic position, this is the place to visit regularly.

Title (or descriptor):	HotJobs
Owner:	Yahoo!, Inc.
URL (Web address):	`http://www.hotjobs.com/`
Rating:	★★

With Yahoo!'s purchase of HotJobs, the site still remains largely oriented toward nonprofessional listings. It is possible that with Yahoo!'s marketing strength, they will be able to change that. In the meantime, you can always check out the advertisement-heavy jobs site if others aren't providing you with enough career opportunities.

Title (or descriptor):	JobLink
Owner:	CenterSite, LLC
URL (Web address):	

`http://www.mentalhelp.net/poc/view_index.php?idx=20`

Rating:	★

The Mental Health Net JobLink is a searchable database of employment opportunities. Its database is culled from online contributions by employers, postings found on mailing lists, and advertisements found on newsgroups and in other publications. It may be beneficial to check once or twice a month for new listings. Since the listings are oriented toward psychology, psychiatry, and the mental health profession in general, position openings may include clinical and academic positions. Listings are categorized by the date they were submitted, with the newest listings appearing first. Mental Health Net also sponsors the other half of the JobLink, which is a listing of individuals' resumes and vitas online. Unfortunately, it doesn't appear that old job postings are regularly removed (jobs more than a year old were found), making it increasingly difficult to search the database and find relevant results.

Title (or descriptor):	MedSearch
Owner:	TMP Worldwide, Inc.
URL (Web address):	`http://www.medsearch.com/`
Rating:	★★★

From the same people who bring you "The Monster Board" (see below) employment resource, this is a resource devoted specifically to medical professionals, which includes the behavioral health care profession. I found a great number of job listings when I did several sample searches. The site is well organized and simple to use. Searches are conducted by entering in a desired geographical location, using a general job category, and any additional keywords you believe applicable. An international job database is available in addition to a U.S. one. It appears that this site uses the same jobs database as Monster.com, but it actually returned fewer results in my sample searches. Perhaps it would be best to simply use Monster.com for job searches.

monster.com
Work. Life. Possibilities.

Title (or descriptor):	The Monster Board
Owner:	TMP Worldwide, Inc.
URL (Web address):	`http://www.monster.com/`
Rating:	★★★★

With a less-than-obvious name, The Monster Board is actually one of the older job databases online. It allows you a number of search options from which to choose, including the simple "Monster Search," which allows you to select a geographical location and general job category (for instance, "Health Care–Psychology"). It returns results nearly instantly. In my sample search, it found 15 related jobs in this category. Using their "keyword" search tool, I found only 6 jobs for a "psychologist" but 120 related to the word "counseling." Your results will obviously vary, but it does offer a large job database and a good selection of search tools. As with most keyword searches online, make sure you use all the possible variants of the word in your query to ensure the most complete search possible. "`Psychology and psychologist`" will get you more results than either one by itself. Some academic jobs are listed in the database as well, and search results are viewed in batches of 10 at a time. Site layout is logical and the graphics are professional and appropriate.

Title (or descriptor):	PsycCareers
Owner:	American Psychological Association
URL (Web address):	`http://www.psyccareers.com/`
Rating:	★★★

The American Psychological Association offers an online version of employment opportunities appearing monthly in the APA's newspaper, *The Monitor*. The employment classified ads are arranged by state and country. A search engine is also available, although it is less than intuitive in its current incarnation, and its search results are somewhat difficult to interpret. These classified ads tend to be oriented toward psychologists and academic positions, as well as the occasional post-doc and internship listing. But some clinical positions usually appear as well. The Web site is fast and easy to navigate; position listings appear as one large file, based on the state or country you select.

Title (or descriptor):	*Psychiatric News* Classifieds
Owner:	American Psychiatric Association
URL (Web address):	
	`http://pn.psychiatryonline.org/misc/classifiedads.shtml`
Rating:	★★★

This site is an online version of the classified section of *Psychiatric News*. It is divided into simple categories by state, country, and position. Unfortunately for you, the publishers have decided to place *all* of the classifieds into one very large file, which will take a few minutes for your Web browser to load. However, once loaded, the file can be easily searched with your browser's "Find" function. *Psychiatric News* is published once every 2 weeks, and this file is updated just as often online. A good location for psychiatrists to check regularly for new employment opportunities.

Title (or descriptor):   *Psychiatric Times* Classifieds

Owner: CME, Inc.

URL (Web address):

    `http://www.psychiatrictimes.com/classified/`

Rating: ★★★

The classified ads from psychiatry's popular monthly magazine, *Psychiatric Times,* are available online, grouped by state (for practice opportunities) or by category, for items such as conferences, fellowships, medical billing, practices for sale, research awards, and other products and services. Simply laid out, the classified ads are easy to browse once a month.

Title (or descriptor):   Social Work and Social Services Jobs Online

Owner: Career Services Office, George Warren Brown School of
                                 Social Work, Washington University

URL (Web address):   `http://gwbweb.wustl.edu/jobs/`

Rating: ★★★

An excellent resource for social workers, jobs are listed by state or country. Hundreds of listings are available through this Web site. Date posted, job title, job location, qualifications of the applicant, salary, job description, a respond-by date, and contact information is provided for each listing.

5

Online Education and Continuing Education Resources

Professional education is available in many forms through the online world. You can find additional information about a university you're thinking of attending or look up more information on the university that employs you. Continuing education programs for clinicians are also becoming available online as an easy and cost-saving alternative to regular continuing education. Learning environments that exist only online—such as online universities—are taking advantage of the technology and the flexibility of the medium that can reach busy people or isolated professionals more easily. Learning through such courses is a new and interesting experience. It may not be right for everyone, but it may fit into your busy schedule more easily than trying to take night classes at the local community college. Or if the nearest university is 100 miles away, this may be a desirable alternative. Nearly all universities and colleges in the world have some sort of Internet presence today, most of them via Web sites.

Online education is very much in its infancy and so you should be aware of the pitfalls and limitations of such programs. Not all may be accredited to award degrees in your state, or even within the United States. Read the fine print carefully before signing up for a 6-month course or 2-year program. If the university or educational organization resides within the United States, a call to the Better Business Bureau in the locale of the university is a very good precaution. They can let you know whether there have been any complaints against the university and if they had been satis-

---

QUICKLY FINDING A UNIVERSITY OR COMPANY ONLINE

While not the most reliable way to find a university, a quick method to locate a particular university's Web site is to simply type in that university's initials as the URL (or Web address), followed by the suffix, ".edu" (which stands for "educational"). For example:

New York University	http://www.nyu.edu/
Ohio State University	http://www.osu.edu/

Sometimes you will need to type in an abbreviation of the university's name:

University of Delaware	http://www.udel.edu/
University of Akron (Ohio)	http://www.uakron.edu/

And for still other universities, you will need to type in the full proper name:

Harvard University	http://www.harvard.edu/
Princeton University	http://www.princeton.edu/

Obviously there is no single way to find a university's home page through this method, but it is a quick and easy thing to try if you're in a hurry. Guides that list all the universities are reviewed below, in case you're not interested in guessing!

Corporate addresses work much the same way, except instead of adding ".edu" to the end of the name, use ".com" (which stands for "commercial"). For example:

Microsoft Corporation	http://www.microsoft.com/
IBM Corporation	http://www.ibm.com/

factorily resolved. Be sure to choose a university and course based on your needs and your comfort level with the technology. If you don't enjoy accessing long reading materials through e-mail, look for an institution that provides Web access to the materials, or vice versa. The right fit between your educational needs and what an institution has to offer is as important in the online world as it is in the real world.

HOW DO I LOCATE A PARTICULAR UNIVERSITY'S PSYCHOLOGY DEPARTMENT OR GRADUATE PROGRAM ONLINE?

There are a number of well-established, reliable sources for finding psychology departments and graduate programs online. One of the easiest and most reliable methods for locating any university or college departmental Web site online is to go to Google (`http://www.google.com/`) and type in the department you are searching for, the word "department," and the name of the university or college enclosed in quotes. For example, if I were searching for the University of Delaware's psychology department, I would type:

```
psychology department "university of delaware"
```

The first entry is the correct one. This foolproof method will find nearly any school's department on the first try. Do you wonder why I did not enclose the words `psychology` and `department` in quotes as well? Because not all schools follow the same naming convention for their departments. Some are known as the "Psychology Department" whereas others are known as the "Department of Psychology." Sometimes it's easier and more reliable to *not* use phrases in a search query when you cannot be certain that phrase is going to be on the page you are looking for. If you don't find the result you are interested in, you can always try one of the resources listed below.

Title (or descriptor):   Links to Other Psychology Departments–Alphabetical Order or by Location

Owner: Hanover College and American Psychological Society

URL (Web address):

http://psych.hanover.edu/Krantz/othera-z.html
(Alphabetical order)

URL (Web address):

http://psych.hanover.edu/Krantz/otherloc.html
(By location)

Rating: ★★★

The alphabetical listing of psychology departments is one very large file, which will take a few minutes to load. The location index (the second URL listed above), however, is not large and is much easier to browse, by state and country. These listings are updated regularly and are about as current as possible with the ever-changing nature of online resource addresses. The Web site sports minimal graphics and is logically arranged. In many cases, where a psychology or related department doesn't yet have a Web site, an e-mail address is listed instead. This allows for online communication. Since this site had psychology departments listed when the Peterson's Education Center didn't, I found it to be more helpful and useful in a quick look to find a psychology department's Web site. If you're looking for a lot more information about a university in particular, though, you might want to check the Peterson's site first.

Title (or descriptor):   Mental Health Related Academic Departments

Owner: Centersite, LLC and Scott Plous

URL (Web address):

http://mentalhelp.net/poc/view_index.php/idx/10
(Geographically)

URL (Web address):

http://www.socialpsychology.org/clinrank.htm
(Graduate Programs in Psychology)

Rating: ★★

A comprehensive guide to psychology, psychiatry, and social work departments and schools online, this guide by Mental Help Net has improved in its breadth and quality of coverage over the years. The second link provides access to a rank-ordered listing of graduate programs in psychology according to the results of a 1995 study by the National Research Council. Stanford University, the University of Michigan–Ann Arbor, Yale University, and UCLA top the list. The Graduate Programs in Psychology listing is provided and maintained by Scott Plous of the Social Psychology Network. This resource's reliability has deteriorated as links have become outdated and no longer appear to be updated.

Title (or descriptor):	Peterson's Education Center
Owner:	The Thompson Corp.
URL (Web address):	`http://www.petersons.com/`
Rating:	★★★

Peterson's is the place to visit when you want to learn a lot more about a university in general: its makeup, general tuition prices, degree offerings, and a host of other useful items. Peterson's is a central clearinghouse of information about college programs, departments, and graduate programs in any major. Offering a comprehensive listing of over 600 graduate programs in psychology and 1,300 undergraduate psychology programs, Peterson's online guide to these programs is unsurpassed. In my sampling, it did, however, miss a few psychology departmental Web pages that are available (and found through the Hanover College/APS listing below). And while it may not be as accurate in its listing of psychology department Web pages, it does offer a current listing of university and college main Web sites. Readers may easily travel to such a central Web site. These then allow you to find the relevant department or program online. Peterson's also offers a useful listing of institutions providing distance learning.

HOW DO I FIND CALENDARS ONLINE THAT LIST PROFESSIONAL EVENTS, CONFERENCES, AND COURSES?

There are several online calendars currently available, which list conferences, courses, workshops, conventions, and events. None is comprehensive. Many calendars exist on small sites, which list only events relevant to their local organization or area. There is no easy or direct way to find these calendars, except by doing a thorough search for them. And because such calendars are often maintained irregularly and updated infrequently, they may be out-of-date and inaccurate.

If you'd like to search for your own profession's calendars, or calendars on specific subtopics not covered below, follow the Step-by-Step instructions.

STEP-BY-STEP INSTRUCTIONS: FINDING A PROFESSIONAL CALENDAR ONLINE

1. Visit a favorite search engine, such as Google:

`http://www.google.com/`

2. Type the following into the search query box to find a social work calendar:

`"social work" calendar —undergraduate —academic —university`

Change the term `"social work"` to `psychology` or `psychiatry` (the quotation marks aren't necessary for single words) to find related calendars.

Specifying `calendar` ensures only those Web sites that reference a calendar appear in the results. Specifying `—undergraduate —academic —university` ensures that you don't retrieve results that are listings of academic courses. These search terms can get you started. Use other terms as needed to limit or expand your search.

Title (or descriptor):	American Psychiatric Association–Schedule of Events
Owner:	American Psychiatric Association
URL (Web address):	`http://www.psych.org/sched_events/`
Rating:	★★

Smaller than CME, Inc.'s site (see below), the APA's Schedule of Events provides members with information on upcoming annual conventions, institutes, and cosponsored events of the American Psychiatric Association. Divided into categories along those divisions, each category offers a fair amount of information on the event itself, especially the larger annual convention and institute. The graphics are professional but may take a while to load. The site's organization is logical and well developed.

Title (or descriptor):	American Psychological Association–Continuing Education Calendar /Conferences
Owner:	American Psychological Association
URL (Web address):	`http://www.apa.org/ce/` (Continuing Education Calendar)

URL (Web address): `http://www.apa.org/about/division/`
`meetings.html` (Conferences)

Rating: ★★★

The American Psychological Association (APA) separates professional meetings from those at which professionals can earn continuing education credits. The Continuing Education Calendar offers a month-by-month listing of dozens of continuing education courses approved by the American Psychological Association. These same listings appear throughout the year in the APA's *Monitor on Psychology,* but here they are searchable online and link to the continuing education provider's Web site. Although the database is large, I found the search engine to be somewhat limiting and requiring the use of Boolean operators. The continuing education search engine was also unable to return results by month and location, so searching for continuing education courses in Maryland in November doesn't currently work. The Conferences section lists information on upcoming cosponsored conferences of the APA, as well as their annual convention (which also has its own section at `http://www.apa.org/convention/`). The site has the usual APA branding and navigation.

Title (or descriptor): At Health Conference Directory

Owner: At Health, Inc.

URL (Web address):

`http://www.athealth.com/practitioner/ceduc/conference.html`

Rating: ★★

A newer directory of continued education offerings available in communities throughout the United States, it is still in its growing stages. Workshops and seminars are listed geographically only and is not currently searchable. The directory has potential with its clean design and its position within the larger At Health professional site.

Title (or descriptor): CME Conferences

Owner: CME, Inc.

URL (Web address): `http://www.mhsource.com/conf/`

Rating: ★★★

Organized by topic, location, and date, this calendar index is directed toward psychiatrists and lists only those conferences sponsored by the large psychiatric continuing education corporation, CME, Inc. An excellent place for psychiatrists to go to keep up-to-date on upcoming conferences and continuing education workshops of relevance to their field or specialty. The site is well designed and easy to navigate, with professional graphics.

Title (or descriptor):   Meetings & Organizations in Behavioral Healthcare & Telehealth

Owner: Myron Pulier, MD

URL (Web address):

    http://www.umdnj.edu/psyevnts/psyjumps.html

Rating: ★★★★

Easily the best and most comprehensive calendar online today, this one covers organizational meetings, events, conferences and courses across disciplines. The calendar is generated through a large and well-maintained database, which means it is up-to-date and accurate. The only drawback to the calendar is that there is no easy way to search it. You have to choose either to view it by a particular month during the year, or by the sponsoring organization's name for the workshop. While both methods are helpful, the ability to search it through keywords would be invaluable and the only improvement on an already great online resource. The site is well organized and has minimal graphics.

ARE THERE APPROVED ONLINE CONTINUING EDUCATION COURSES THAT I CAN TAKE?

The world of online continuing education offerings has undergone a shake-up in recent years, with providers either shutting down or redesigning their efforts. Too few professionals signed up for these courses to make them viable businesses. Some programs are sticking it out, however, and others are trying more integrated and larger multimedia approaches.

Continuing education courses online typically take three forms—text-based, discussion-based, and multimedia. Text-based courses typically take a tutorial format. Information is organized on a course Web page with related links to other, independent Web sites. The user reads the information at their leisure and takes a quiz at the end to test for knowledge and gain their continuing education credit. This is the least innovate online course method, similar to traditional home-based continuing education. The major difference is that the participant reads from a computer screen rather than paper.

Discussion-based courses revolve around an expert-led professional discussion, generally in an online private, closed space such as a mailing list. Participants contribute to the discussion in an interactive learning process. This is more innovative than text-based courses, as it leverages community technologies to offer a unique way of learning.

The third type of online course is the most innovative of them all. It leverages the full capabilities of the Internet's multimedia potential by integrating audio, video, a slide presentation, and discussion. The range of multimedia offerings online varies. Some services offer audio and synchronized slide presentations, with an asynchronous discussion forum. Others offer a synchronous, classroomlike environment with audio, a slide presentation, and real time chat.

Title (or descriptor):	At Health e-Campus
Owner:	At Health, Inc.
URL (Web address):	`http://www.athealthce.com/`
Rating:	★★★

At Health offers a strong continuing education offering of more than 4 dozen courses. Most of the courses are available online in a simple format—read an article, answer a few questions in a quiz, and get one or two continuing education courses that count toward a professional's license upkeep. Home study courses have been doing this for years, and its translation online works well for the time-challenged, harried professional. Because the courses are not interactive, professionals can take courses at their leisure, taking as much time as they need to complete them. Some additional courses are available via more traditional methods, such as audio and videotape.

Most courses are approved for professional continuing education credit by the American Psychological Association, the Association of Social Work Boards, and the National Board for Certified Counselors. Prices vary from $10 to $30 per credit hour. The course catalog provides a complete list of courses arranged within topical categories, such as Attention Deficit Disorder, Childhood Disorders, Depression,

SENDING CREDIT CARD INFORMATION ONLINE

Never send credit card information online unless you encrypt it first. There are two common ways to encrypt (or encode information to prevent easy access to it, except by the authorized recipient) information online: (1) a special encryption program (such as Pretty Good Privacy programs) to use through e-mail; or (2) a Web site's encryption software, which is activated automatically by your Web browser. The first option is more complicated than I can go into here. The second option is what you will most often come across while browsing the Web.

A Web site supports encryption of your credit card information when your browser lets you know it has entered a "secure" page on a Web site. This usually includes a visual cue in the browser (e.g., in Netscape Navigator, the small picture of an open lock or broken key in the lower left-hand corner of the browser window will become a closed, highlighted lock or a whole key). It may also include a warning box that is automatically displayed when you enter or leave the secure area on the Web site.

Web developers who are concerned about your privacy and security of your financial information will be aware of these issues and let you know whether they support encryption of your credit card information. If they do not, *do not enter your credit card information online*. When in doubt, don't do it. A telephone number is usually provided as an alternative method of paying for the product or service. Do not even consider using a Web site that requests credit card information and that isn't aware of these basic security measures.

Ethics, Pharmacology, Practice Digests, and Risk Management, among others. By clicking on a course's title, you learn more about the course instructor, the course's learning objectives, a course description and syllabus, cost, and continuing education credit, if available. The help section is complete and answered all of my questions. The site even includes a helpful demonstration that walks you through choosing a course, taking it, how the online testing works, how to communicate with course instructors, and more. At Health offers a well thought-out offering that gives professionals a reliable choice for receiving online continuing education at their leisure.

Title (or descriptor):   Interactive Testing in Psychiatry

Owner: New York University Department of Psychiatry and the New University Post-Graduate Medical School

URL (Web address):

`http://www.mrcr4.med.nyu.edu/Psych/itp.html`

Rating: ★★★

Access restrictions: Fees: $20.00/credit hour (up to 7 hours available)

This very user-friendly program allows you to answer Board-style questions just by clicking on buttons. The Web site automatically calculates your score and can give you the correct answer to every question. Seven modules are available, consisting of 30 questions each. Individuals are welcome to take the modules for free, or they can apply for continuing education credit in psychiatry by submitting a $20.00 fee for each module. There are, however, no online reading materials to consult, nor are there any Web links to additional reference materials. All that is available to readers is a "References" category, which lists books for further reading (and contains the answers to the questions in each module).

Modules are arranged in no particular order, nor are the questions contained within each module. Questions cover the full breadth of psychiatry, but tend to focus

on pharmacology and diagnosis.

Title (or descriptor):	PsyBC
Owner:	Psy Broadcasting Corporation
URL (Web address):	`http://www.psybc.com/`
Rating:	★★★★
Access restrictions:	Fees: $7.50/credit hour (courses typically range from 6 to 8 credit hours)

The Psy Broadcasting Corporation is a Web site offering a service akin to a professional mailing where the participants are charged to listen in on the conversation. The "broadcasting" referred to in the name is simply the use of a mailing list to carry on a conversation among panels of selected professionals in certain fields, such as cognitive behavioral therapy, mood disorders, and psychopharmacology. PsyBC is a reliable service that has come into its own over the years, providing an array of online courses in multiple formats at reasonable prices.

WHERE DO I LOOK TO FIND REGULAR UNIVERSITY PROGRAMS AND COURSES OFFERED ONLINE?

This idea, which is commonly termed "distance learning," has been around for decades. Many people confuse such educational programs with universities or institutions that just hand out degrees for a fee ("degree mills"). Most distance-learning institutions, though, are not degree mills and many are associated with a larger, well-known university to ensure quality and standards. As recommended at the start of this chapter, check out an institution through the Better Business Bureau before signing up for courses. If you're still wary, ask for references from individuals who have already completed courses and e-mail them asking about their experiences. Such precautions can help reduce the possibility of disappointment.

Searching Guides to Online Education

The best way to find out more about online education is by browsing through the guides listed below and sample some of the Web-site offerings by the many institutions listed.

Title (descriptor):	Open Directory Project: Distance Learning
Owner:	Netscape
URL:	

```
http://dmoz.org/Reference/Education/Distance_Learning/
```

Rating:	★★★

Similar to Yahoo!'s directory listing of distance learning opportunities, the Open Directory Project offers similar choices and categories. As with all of the Open Directory Project, the site is quick to load and offers simple graphics, and, refreshingly, no banner advertising.

Title (descriptor):	Peterson's Education Center
Owner:	The Thompson Corp.

URL:

> http://www.petersons.com/distancelearning/

Rating: ★★★

Please see the full review of Peterson's earlier in this section.

Title (descriptor):   Psychology Ed-X Course Listing

Owner: Ed-X, LLC

URL:

> http://www.ed-x.com/courselistings/psychology.asp

Rating: ★★★

Ed-X provides listings of courses available over the Internet from dozens of different universities and educational institutions. Offering a convenient interface that allows the user to choose from different subfields within psychology (such as clinical, abnormal, child and adolescent, sports psychology, etc.), it provides an index of numerous courses offered within each category, along with the offering institution's name and geographical location. Clicking on a course title takes you to that institution's course page, which provides in-depth, detailed information about the course, its cost, and how it's provided online.

Title (or descriptor):   Yahoo! Education: Distance Learning

Owner: Yahoo!, Inc.

URL (Web address):

> http://www.yahoo.com/Education/Distance_Learning/

Rating: ★★★

Yahoo! is one of the easier places to find a distance learning resource among the hundreds listed within this category. Check under both the "Colleges and Universities" category as well as the "On-Line Teaching and Learning" category. Yahoo!'s descriptions are sometimes less than informative, but under the "Colleges and Universities" category, keep a lookout for those that offer courses online through the Internet or e-mail. Many such programs are available, and they cover a multitude of topics ranging from the expected (computer programming) to those relevant to mental health professionals (health, mental health, and social welfare). Like all of Yahoo!, the site is quick to load and offers simple graphics (and your typical banner advertising, which helps pay the bills).

Visiting Select University Web Sites

I've chosen just a few of the multitude of institutions that now offer some sort of education online. These sites are listed here just to give you a general idea of the types of experiences you can expect to have when enrolling in an online university. I do not personally endorse any of these sites, nor have I taken any of their courses, so I cannot vouch for their usefulness or quality; therefore rating scores have been omitted in this section.

Title (or descriptor):	Foothill Global Access
Owner:	Foothill College
URL (Web address):	`http://www.foothillglobalaccess.org/`
Access restrictions:	Yes; fee unpublished

Unlike some other institutions that offer online courses, Foothill College simply makes available online many of its regular undergraduate courses. The program is not organized in any logical way to obtain a specific degree. As at the University of Phoenix, courses are not self-directed or open-ended; they start and end at specific times throughout the year, based on a quarter schedule (fall, winter, spring, and summer). Teaching is done entirely through group e-mail (a mailing list), as are testing and other regular class activities. The course credit is as transferable as regular course credit to other universities, the college claims, but that will largely be dependent on the university to which you want to transfer the credit. Each class is taught by a regular instructor, and courses are offered on a wide variety of subjects ranging from computers and art, to economics and business. The Web site offers little information beyond the basics and leaves a lot of obvious questions unanswered.

Title (or descriptor):	Nova Southeastern University Distance Education
Owner:	Nova Southeastern University
URL (Web address):	`http://www.nova.edu/cwis/disted/`
Access restrictions:	Yes; fees variable

Nova Southeastern University is one of the pioneers in distance education, having been in the business since 1972 and offering courses online since 1983. They use a variety of technologies and formats, from video and audio conferencing in regular remote classrooms, to purely Internet-based courses. The university offers a wide range of degree program options, ranging from a master of medical science and graduate teacher education programs to business and professional management and graduate degrees in computer sciences. The site offers a great deal of useful information about the programs, but individual schools within the university are responsible for maintaining their own sites. This leads to a greater degree of variability in the information and design, which makes it more difficult than necessary to find what you need.

Title (or descriptor):	At Health e-Campus
Owner:	At Health, Inc.
URL (Web address):	`http://www.athealthce.com/`
Access restrictions:	Yes; fees range from $10 to $80 per course

At Health has a large course catalog offering over 100 courses, about half of which are available online (the others are available through books, audio-, or videocassettes). Because At Health acts as a course aggregator, approved continuing education credit for each mental health profession varies from course to course. But with the wide variety of courses offered, At Health is likely to have something to offer most professionals in search of online continuing education.

Title (or descriptor):	University of Phoenix Online
Owner:	University of Phoenix
URL (Web address):	`http://online.phoenix.edu`
Access restrictions:	$410/credit hour for graduate courses and $335/credit hour for undergraduate courses

One of the leading online institutions, the University of Phoenix offers Bachelor of Science degree programs in business/administration, business/information systems, business/management; Master of Arts in organizational management; Master of Business Administration, Master of Business Administration/Technology Management, and Master of Business Administration/Global Management. The Web site is fast and offers professional graphics as well as copious information, including a fre-

quently asked questions file (also called an "FAQ"), which answered all of my immediate questions. This institution appears to take education seriously. It lets prospective students know that it will take anywhere from 2 to 3 years to complete a program. Course tuition is also not cheap; comparable community college courses
within your local area probably cost much less. Unlike other online institutions, the
courses are not self-paced or open-ended; they are scheduled much like regular real-
world classes. Most of the work is done through reading assigned texts, either offline
or through the university's online library. It all appears to be well organized and
many students have already successfully completed the programs.

Title (or descriptor):   World Wide Learn

Owner: World Wide Learn

URL (Web address):

```
http://www.worldwidelearn.com/continuing-education/
psychologists-cme.htm
```

World Wide Learn provides a fairly up-to-date directory of continuing education
courses for psychologists. It includes additional entries not found in this chapter, although not all of the providers listed had working links.

6

Networking with Other Professionals Online

The Internet allows professionals to keep in touch with others around the world at a fraction of the cost of regular telephone use, and in a much more timely manner than going through the postal service. The online tools range from the mundane (e-mail directories) to cutting-edge technology (Internet telephone and videoconferencing, discussed in Chapter 10). This chapter examines how to participate in online case conferences and ongoing discussion groups with other professionals, how to quickly find someone's e-mail address, and how to track down other professionals conducting particular kinds of research.

Professional discussion areas are among the most popular and widely used online resources. Such discussions usually take place through mailing lists, which are basically a form of group electronic mail. In these forums, like-minded clinicians and researchers can discuss specific issues on a wide range of professional topics. Most such discussion areas are focused on specific topic areas, such as forensic psychology, clinical psychology, clinical social work, psychopharmacology, and so forth. Professionals may use such forums for reading or posting announcements of workshops, conferences, or employment; engaging in theoretical, research-oriented, or clinical discussions; and exchanging information about valuable books, journal references, or online resources that may benefit other professionals. It is in these kinds of discussion areas where most professionals tend to gather online and probably the first area you should go to if you're new online. Why? Because most of these discussion areas are mailing lists, which are simple to subscribe to and easy to use. These will be covered later in this chapter.

An additional use of many discussion areas online is the presentation of a formal or informal case conference. I will illustrate this example in depth, because it is one of the most useful to a wide variety of practitioners.

WHERE CAN I PARTICIPATE IN ONLINE CASE CONFERENCES?

There are many areas online where you can participate in a case conference. Before I discuss specific online resources, however, I will first present an overview of the purpose of online case conferences. Case conferences exist online for a number of the same reasons they do in the real world. First and foremost, they allow professionals to present current cases that may be presenting some difficulty in treatment. The difficulty may arise because of a unique or rare disorder, the clinician's lack of experience in treating a particular type of disorder, or an abnormal presentation of a disorder, which the therapist would like to gain some additional insight on and clarify his or her own conceptualization of it. When presenting cases, clinicians usually discuss explicitly their reasons for asking for input on the case. Second, professionals will also present cases for comment when they have treated a particularly difficult case. By sharing the case and treatment approach, other professionals may gain some benefit from the ensuing discussion. Third, clinicians who are isolated from their colleagues (for instance, due to working in an independent practice or in remote or rural areas) benefit from case conferences, keeping them in touch with current trends in treatment and outcomes. There are many additional benefits (such as research and training) in case conferences, but these are the central ones. As discussed in Chapter 8, professionals should exercise the same care when presenting cases in any online forum as they would in real life. Identifying information should be omitted or changed enough so that someone who may be reading the case presentation and know the person being presented could not easily identify that person through your online description.

Types of Online Case Conferences

Case conferences online are of two basic types: formal and informal. In formal case conferences, invited faculty—usually well-known figures in their particular subspecialty area—present a difficult case from their history. Other invited faculty are then encouraged to comment on aspects of the case from their particular theoretical perspectives. Other professionals may participate in the ensuing discussion or simply sit back and read it as it enfolds. These formal presentations are most often made in a Web-based discussion area, because the messages don't expire and the discussion threads are simple to follow and read. This easily allows newcomers to "get up to speed" on the discussion thus far. There is no reason these presentations can't be made in a live, interactive chat group online, or through some related medium such as audio or video, except that such technologies are not as well known as the Web or e-mail are to most professionals or may not be readily available to them.

Informal case discussions are far more prevalent. They often take place through mailing lists rather than in Web-based discussion areas. Mailing lists are simple; the e-mail technology involved is available to anyone online. You must first sign up or "subscribe" to a mailing list, but this is easy to do for most people (see the "Step-by-Step: Subscribing to a Mailing List" on page 112). In an informal case presentation, a professional who has subscribed to the particular mailing list simply sends an e-mail to the list describing the patient or client (keeping confidentiality in mind), his presenting problem, a little bit about his background and relevant personal history, and treatment to date. The clinician may also talk about her conceptualization of the case before getting feedback from other professionals, or she may decide to withhold it until after she has elicited others' opinions. Additional questions may be asked of the professional who presents the case online, and they are usually quickly answered.

The elegance and beauty of case conferences online is that opinions come from many different people with vastly different backgrounds, professional orientations, and experiences from around the world. A wealth of knowledge and information exists in these online discussion areas that cannot exist easily or often in the real world. This is one of the best examples of an online experience that is actually quantitatively and qualitatively better than a similar experience in the real world. Every organization I have worked in as a clinician has held case conferences. But most organizations are closed systems; new information rarely permeates the outer "walls" that have been built up over years within the organization. Universities and graduate schools can often be notable exceptions, when the programs are larger and encourage diversity within their clinical tracks.

Online case conferences suffer no such limitations because the online world is inherently an open system. There is an easy experiment you can conduct to test this observation. Present the same case both to your colleagues in a staff meeting or case conference, and also to one of the online conferences. Ask for treatment suggestions and conceptualizations. I will bet that you will receive a much more diverse and rich response from those individuals in the online conference than from your real-world colleagues.

So where do you find these conferences? There is one Web site I am aware of that offers formal presentations, and that is Behavior OnLine (described in detail below). Formal case presentations in the real world are often made in association with universities, so you might also keep tabs on schools that have a strong online presence to see if they offer case conferences. (Quite frankly, I don't know of any who currently do.) Informal case conferences exist most often on professionally oriented mailing lists. For instance, the clinical psychologists mailing list (listed under "Psychologists, Clinical" on page 139) sometimes features discussions among psychologists about specific cases.

The next section gives details on mailing lists and includes how to find those that may have informal case conferences. I also keep an index of such lists on my Web site, PsychCentral.com.

A Formal Case Conference

Title (or descriptor):	Behavior OnLine
Owner:	Behavior OnLine
URL (Web address):	`http://www.behavior.net/`
Rating:	★★★★

Behavior OnLine, the online gathering place for professionals, started out as a small, well-designed Web site that featured conversations (actually, interviews) with five well-known professionals within their specific subspecialty areas. Some of these professionals also went on to participate in ongoing discussion forums on the same site. Behavior OnLine expanded them further and made use of their unique features and attributes. These include the ability to keep discussions around for as long as they remain relevant, as well as offering a format that makes reading easy and logical: Through a process called "threading," responses to an original message appear directly under that first message.

Behavior OnLine launched its first formal case conference in June of 1996 and has since followed up with a handful of additional presentations. Invited faculty present their cases, and a lively and interesting discussion then ensues. Participants may simply follow along or offer their own insights and opinions on the presented case.

The Web site itself, which has not been redesigned in years, retains a simple yet elegant layout and design. The lack of updating to newer and more feature-laden discussion forum software is the only drawback to Behavior OnLine. The forum software currently in use doesn't allow simple options such as a regular membership login and profile, saving user preferences, and signature files. I am an associate editor with Behavior Online.

WHERE DO I FIND TOPIC-ORIENTED DISCUSSIONS WITH OTHER PROFESSIONALS ONLINE?

Mailing List Discussions

Naturally, case conferences are just one aspect of using discussion forums online. There are dozens of professional mailing lists from which to choose, all of which may be relevant to you as a professional, depending on area of expertise or interest. While I have endeavored to list all I know of below, I am certain that more have been added since this book went to press. That is why by using such resources as Liszt and Psych Central, you can easily to identify newer mailing lists that may not appear here. As reviewed in Chapter 2, these resources specialize in helping you find lists in your areas of interest.

Mailing lists are the most popular way for professionals to network with one another online, largely because of their ease of use. Many professional mailing lists are *credentialed*, which means you might have to first submit proof of your professional status before the facilitators will allow you to subscribe. This protects the professionals currently subscribed to the list from off-topic conversations from nonprofessionals; it ensures that you are who you say you are. It is relatively easy for unscrupulous individuals to pretend they are someone else online or pretend to expertise and credentials they don't have. Most professional mailing lists are also *closed*. A closed list means that only subscribers to the list can actually send messages to it. Open mailing lists, on the other hand, allow even nonsubscribers to post to the list. The advantage of a closed mailing list is that it won't often be used for off-topic advertisements. Some professionals still post the occasional employment opportunity or conference announcement, but these notices are usually relevant to the list's topic and occur so rarely that it is not bothersome. Closed mailing lists are just as easy to join as open mailing lists, and they are the preferred standard in the online world for professional discussions.

Mailing lists, like newsgroups, may also be moderated. "Moderated" means that before an article is published to the list, a human being (the "moderator") approves its content. This ensures that only those articles that are on-topic for that particular mailing list make it out to the hundreds of other list members. Most professional mailing lists are not moderated because they are closed. The list owner can ensure only professionals subscribe to their list at the outset, which then makes a task like moderating largely unnecessary.

Mailing lists tend to be subject-specific, and those oriented toward mental health professionals are no different. A list for professional discussion of addictions is different from the one for the discussion of affective disorders; some topics may even have multiple lists. List quality and traffic (how much e-mail you will receive each day from the list) varies greatly. My suggestion is that you subscribe to one list at a time and see if it suits you in terms of quality and traffic. Allow a week or two to go by before you make your decision.

If you can't locate a mailing list on a topic that interests you, you may want to consider starting one on your own. Mailing lists are relatively easy to create and simple to maintain in most cases. Many well-equipped Internet Service Providers have the facilities to allow you to host a mailing list or two if you'd like. For further information on this topic, speak to a customer service representative at your Internet Service Provider.

An alternative to creating a new mailing list through your service provider is to use one of the many free and low-cost mailing list serv-

MAILING LIST ETIQUETTE

Mailing list etiquette varies from forum to forum. On low-traffic, smaller lists, it is often considered polite to introduce yourself after you have subscribed, telling list members a bit about your background and interest in the list's topic. High-volume lists frown on such introductions, since there is already so much (and often times, too much!) e-mail being exchanged on the list. If you're unsure what to do, you can always privately e-mail the list's owner and ask.

Never send mailing list commands (e.g., subscribe or unsubscribe) to the list address! They don't work if you send them to the wrong address and you end up annoying hundreds of other subscribers on the list. That's why I've included *all the information* you will need to both subscribe and unsubscribe from a mailing list. I have also hunted down the list's description and list owner's name and e-mail address so if you have any further questions about the list, you can write that person directly.

Once subscribed to a mailing list, you will start receiving e-mail messages that are distributed to everyone on the list. Typically when you want to reply to a message on a list, you just choose your e-mail software's "Reply" feature. Your response will usually automatically be sent to every other member on the list as well. It is a good idea to differentiate between replies you'd like to send to the entire list (hundreds of people) and those you'd like to send only to the original author of a message (e.g., a regular, private e-mail). It is always a good idea, therefore, to double-check the "To:" line of your reply e-mail to ensure it is being sent to the correct addressee.

STEP-BY-STEP: SUBSCRIBING TO A MAILING LIST

Many mailing lists available online today offer two ways to subscribe—through the traditional method (listed below) or through the mailing list's Web site. If a mailing list is hosted by a large organization or company (such as the American Psychological Association, Yahoo! or Topica), they will often have a Web site that provides direct access to the mailing list's message archive and one-click options to subscribe or unsubscribe from the list.

1. Create a new e-mail message. Ensure the message is sent as *plain text,* not HTML. Turn off any fancy stationary options.

2. Address it to the e-mail address in the "Commands to:" listed below for that specific mailing list.

3. Don't fill in anything for the "Subject" of your e-mail message (or use a single space if your e-mail software requires the subject line to be filled in).

4. In the body of your e-mail, write *exactly* what is listed below in the "Subscribe" field for that mailing list. This is the command you use to tell the mailing list software to add you to the list.

5. If needed, as noted in each listing below, replace the phrase "Your-name" with your actual name (e.g., `John Grohol`); or, alternatively, replace the phrase "Your-email-address" with your actual e-mail address (e.g., `grohol@netscape.com`). If neither is noted in the listing, then the subscription command will look simply like "subscribe name-of-mailing-list" (without the quotes).

6. Do not write anything else in the e-mail.

7. Send the e-mail and wait for an automated reply, which should confirm your subscription request within 24 hours. Some mailing lists may also require you to respond to the automated reply to confirm your subscription. Instructions for doing so are included in the automated reply if this is required.

ice providers. Free service providers include Yahoo! (`http://www.yahoogroups.com/`) and Topica (`http://www.topica.com/`). These are full-service providers, offering your mailing list a Web page to host archives and a description of the list, as well as a simple Web-based interface for both your subscribers and administrative functions. But nothing in life is truly free; services typically place advertising in every message sent

UNDERSTANDING MAILING LIST RESOURCE HEADINGS

Title (or descriptor): Name or description of the mailing list.

Web site: `http://psychcentral.com/`
Some mailing lists also have Web sites, which can give you additional information about the list. The Web site may also house the list's archives. This heading only appears when a mailing list has a known Web site.

Commands to: `listserv@nowhere.com`
This is the e-mail address to which you address all of your subscribe and unsubscribe requests.

Subscribe: `subscribe Listname Your-name`
This is the subscribe command you place in the body of your e-mail message, substituting "Your-name" or "Your-email-address" with the appropriate name or address. The "Listname" is the proper name of the mailing list.

Unsubscribe: `unsubscribe Listname`
This is the unsubscribe command you place in the body of your e-mail message. Notice you *do not* include your name or e-mail address in this request.

List: `Listname@nowhere.com`
This is the address of the mailing list itself, to which you may send your messages to get distributed to all the list's subscribers after you have become a member of the list.

List owner: John Smith (E-mail: `johnsmith@nowhere.com`)
This is the person responsible for maintaining the list and helping people subscribe and unsubscribe. He or she may also participate in and lead the list's discussion.

to the list in order to offset the costs of running the service. For a small monthly fee, these ads can be removed. Because it is easier than ever to create one of these lists, I strongly encourage you to consider starting a mailing list on a professional topic of interest to you.

Once you have subscribed to a mailing list, you will remain subscribed to it and continue receiving e-mail from the list for as long as it exists. For any of a number of reasons (e.g., you may be receiving too much e-mail from the list, you are changing e-mail accounts, you are going on vacation), you may wish to unsubscribe from that mailing list. You follow the same steps you used to subscribe to the list, except you substitute the "unsub-

STEP-BY-STEP: UNSUBSCRIBING FROM A MAILING LIST

1. Create a new e-mail message. Ensure the message is sent as *plain text,* not HTML. Turn off any fancy stationary options.

2. Address it to the e-mail address in the "Commands to:" listed below for that specific mailing list.

3. Don't fill in anything for the "Subject" of your e-mail message (or use a single space if your e-mail software requires the subject line to be filled in).

4. In the body of your e-mail, write *exactly* what is in the "Unsubscribe" field for that mailing list. This is the command you use to tell the mailing list software to remove you from the list.

5. Do not write anything else in the e-mail.

6. Send the e-mail and wait for a reply e-mail, which should confirm your unsubscription request within 24 hours. If you have any difficulties, contact the list owner directly through his or her own e-mail address.

7. If you ever lose the unsubscription instructions to a particular list that you are subscribed to, try this handy tip:

    A. Note the name of the mailing list and its domain. This is typically the e-mail address that appears in the "To:" line of e-mail sent to the list. For example, a list's "To:" line might read "To: `medwebmasters-L@listserv.acor.org`." Everything before the "@" sign is the mailing list's name, and everything after the "@" sign is the list's domain. In this case, the name of the list is "medwebmasters-L" and its domain is "acor.org."

scribe" command for the "subscribe" command (see the box, "Unsubscribing from a Mailing List").

Below, I've given a brief summary description of some relevant and interesting mailing lists. The descriptions are gleaned from the list's owner or publicly available information. Sample topics may also be included in the description. These may not be the topics currently under discussion on the list but are *examples* of topics that *may* be discussed on it. Mailing

B. Compose a new e-mail message and address it to the following three addresses:

```
listserv@domain.name
listproc@domain.name
majordomo@domain.name
nameoflist-unsubscribe@domain.name
```

Replace "domain.name" with the list's actual domain. In the example from above, we would compose our e-mail to the following three addresses:

```
listserv@listserv.acor.org
listproc@listserv.acor.org
majordomo@listserv.acor.org
medwebmasters-L-unsubscribe@listserv.acor.org
```

C. Leave the subject line of the e-mail message blank.

D. In the body of your e-mail message, write:

```
unsubscribe listname
```

where "listname" is the name of the list we discovered in step A. In the example from above, this would look like:

```
unsubscribe medwebmasters-L
```

E. Send the e-mail message.

What will now happen is that your e-mail will be sent to all three e-mail addresses. More than likely, two of them will be invalid and the e-mail will be returned to you as "undeliverable." Delete those messages when they arrive. But one of those e-mails you sent will be successful in unsubscribing you from the mailing list 99.99 percent of the time. I have never had this trick fail. Many mailing lists have associated Web sites, such as those hosted by Yahoo! Groups and Topica. You can also unsubscribe yourself from a list by visiting the mailing list's Web site.

list addresses change from time to time (although usually not too often). If you have difficulty with any of the addresses below, check the book's Web site for a complete up-to-date listing of these addresses (http://www.insidemh.com/), or consult the updated lists at Psych Central (http://psychcentral.com/). Nearly all of the mailing lists discussed below are maintained by professionals, with some maintained by *the* leading figures within the field. Individuals who maintain mailing lists are referred to as "list owners" because they "own" the list. These people are responsible for creating the list in the first place and are typically in charge of ongoing administration as well. If you have any questions or problems subscribing to a mailing list below, the list owner can often help you properly subscribe to the list.

Professional Mailing Lists

Title (or descriptor):	Addiction Medicine
Commands to:	`listserv@maelstrom.stjohns.edu`
Subscribe:	`subscribe ADD_MED Your-name`
Unsubscribe:	`unsubscribe ADD_MED`
List:	`ADD_MED@maelstrom.stjohns.edu`
List owner:	John French (E-mail: `john.french@verizon.net`)

A closed scientific discussion list for health professionals and students interested in a discussion on research, diagnosis, and treatment of dependence on psychoactive substances (including alcohol), dual diagnosis, and other behaviors that can be viewed by an addictive model.

Title (or descriptor):	Addictions
Commands to:	`listserv@listserv.kent.edu`
Subscribe:	`subscribe Addict-L Your-name`
Unsubscribe:	`unsubscribe Addict-L`
List:	`addict-L@listserv.kent.edu`

A list for the academic and scholarly discussion of addiction related topics. The focus of the professional discussion is often on sexual, co-addiction, eating, alcohol/drug addiction, research methodology and outcome. Recovery issues are also appropriate.

Title (or descriptor):	Affective Disorders
Commands to:	`listserv@maelstrom.stjohns.edu`
Subscribe:	`subscribe AFFECTD Your-name`
Unsubscribe:	`unsubscribe AFFECTD`
List:	`AFFECTD@maelstrom.stjohns.edu`
List owner:	Steven Dubovsky (E-mail: `steven.dubovsky@uchsc.edu`)

A forum for discourse on all aspects of affective disorders, including depression, mood, and bipolar disorders.

Title (or descriptor):	American Association of Applied and Preventive Psychology (AAAPP)
Commands to:	`listserv@LSV.UKY.EDU`
Subscribe:	`subscribe AAAPP Your-name`
Unsubscribe:	`unsubscribe AAAPP`
List:	`AAAPP@LSV.UKY.EDU`
List owner:	Various (E-mail: `AAAPP-request@LSV.UKY.EDU`)

For members of the American Association of Applied and Preventive Psychology (AAAPP).

Title (or descriptor):	Anxiety Disorders
Commands to:	`listserv@maelstrom.stjohns.edu`
Subscribe:	`subscribe ANX-DIS Your-name`
Unsubscribe:	`unsubscribe ANX-DIS`
List:	`ANX-DIS@maelstrom.stjohns.edu`
List owner:	Charles Figley (E-mail: `cfigley@garnet.acns.fsu.edu`)

A scholary forum for mental health professionals to discuss anxiety disorders.

Title (or descriptor):   Applied Behavioral Analysis

Web site:

    `http://groups.yahoo.com/group/ABA-social-behavior/`

Subscribe:

    `ABA-social-behavior-subscribe@yahoogroups.com`

Unsubscribe:

    `ABA-social-behavior-unsubscribe@yahoogroups.com`

List: `ABA-social-behavior@yahoogroups.com`

A forum for support and strategies, including applied behavioral analysis (ABA) approaches, to address the unique social and behavioral deficits of those diagnosed with high-functioning forms of autistic spectrum disorders, including Asperger's disorder.

Title (or descriptor):   Attachment Issues

Commands to: `listserv@maelstrom.stjohns.edu`

Subscribe: `subscribe attach Your-name`

Unsubscribe: `unsubscribe attach`

List: `attach@maelstrom.stjohns.edu`

List owner: Chuck Hollister (E-mail: `gauguin@ix.netcom.com`)

                   Cherie Rawlins (E-mail: `veronica2@telus.net`)

This list emphasizes socio-affective and defensive processes, as well as unconscious representations. Discussion includes Bowlby–Ainsworth theory of attachment.

Title (or descriptor):   Behavioral Neuroscience News

Web site:

    `http://groups.yahoo.com/group/BehavioralNeuroscience/`

Subscribe:

    `BehavioralNeuroscience-subscribe@yahoogroups.com`

Unsubscribe:

    `BehavioralNeuroscience-unsubscribe@yahoogroups.com`

List: `BehavioralNeuroscience@yahoogroups.com`

This is an announcement-only mailing list that shares articles members find on the Internet concerning biological psychology and behavioral neuroscience. The list is intended to help interested professionals and students keep up with the latest developments in the field.

Title (or descriptor):   Behavioral School Psychology

Web site:

> `http://groups.yahoo.com/group/NASP-IG-BehavioralSP/`

Subscribe:

> `NASP-IG-BehavioralSP-subscribe@yahoogroups.com`

Unsubscribe:

> `NASP-IG-BehavioralSP-unsubscribe@yahoogroups.com`

List: `NASP-IG-BehavioralSP@yahoogroups.com`

A professional forum sponsored by the National Association of School Psychologists (`http://www.nasponline.org/`) for the discussion of behavioral school psychology.

Title (or descriptor):   Behavioral Science

Web site: `http://groups.yahoo.com/group/behscience/`

Subscribe: `behscience-subscribe@yahoogroups.com`

Unsubscribe: `behscience-unsubscribe@yahoogroups.com`

List: `behscience@yahoogroups.com`

This active group seeks to improve behavioral scientists' overall level of satisfaction with their roles in family practice settings through peer support, mentoring, curriculum development, and sharing resources and information. It hopes to promote the integration of the behavioral sciences in family medicine practice and keep group members abreast of the latest news and developments in the field.

Title (or descriptor):   Bodywork Practitioners

Web site: `http://groups.yahoo.com/group/Body_Work/`

Subscribe: `Body_Work-subscribe@yahoogroups.com`

Unsubscribe: `Body_Work-unsubscribe@yahoogroups.com`

List: `Body_Work@yahoogroups.com`

For the professional discussion of bodywork therapies, such as Swedish massage, Trager approach, trigger point therapy, Rolfing, polarity therapy, Reiki, reflexology, Alexander technique, Jin Shin Do, acupuncture, and Shiatsu. Physical therapy and training issues are also appropriate topics.

Title (or descriptor):   Business Consultation for Professionals (PsyBUS)

Web site:

   `http://telehealth.net/subscribe/psybus.html`

Commands to: `listserv@maelstrom.stjohns.edu`

Subscribe: `subscribe PsyBUS Your-name`

Unsubscribe: `unsubscribe PsyBUS`

List: `PsyBUS@maelstrom.stjohns.edu`

List owner: Marlene Maheu (E-mail: `drm@cybertowers.com`)

This list facilitates a discussion among practicing psychotherapists across disciplines interested in the development and marketing of practice-related products and services. There are no fees to join or participate.

Title (or descriptor):   Child Sexual Abuse Prevention

Web site: `http://groups.yahoo.com/group/csap/`

Subscribe: `csap-subscribe@yahoogroups.com`

Unsubscribe: `csap-unsubscribe@yahoogroups.com`

List: `csap@yahoogroups.com`

List owner: Alisa Klein (E-mail: `aklein@stopitnow.org`)

This forum is for professional discussion about the prevention of child sexual abuse. It is for the exchange of ideas, research, and other professional material, and timely information about events and meetings related to the prevention of child sexual abuse.

Title (or descriptor):	Clinical Psychophysiology and Biofeedback
Commands to:	`majordomo@listp.apa.org`
Subscribe:	`subscribe PSYPHY`
Unsubscribe:	`unsubscribe PSYPHY`
List:	`PSYPHY@listp.apa.org`
List owner:	Arnon Rolnick (E-mail: `telhome@netvision.net.il`)

This forum is for the discussion of all aspects of psychophysiology and biofeedback. This includes techniques and treatment methods in the fields of medicine, psychology, psychiatry, social work, education, and sports medicine.

Title (or descriptor): Cognitive Neuroscience

Web site:

`http://groups.yahoo.com/group/cognitiveneuroscienceforum/`

Subscribe:

`cognitiveneuroscienceforum-subscribe@yahoogroups.com`

Unsubscribe:

`cognitiveneuroscienceforum-unsubscribe@yahoogroups.com`

List:

`cognitiveneuroscienceforum@yahoogroups.com`

This forum, open to both researchers and nonresearchers, offers lively discussion on the nature of intelligence, behavior, sleep, and the role of the arts and sciences in relation to our increasing knowledge of the brain's makeup and neurology.

Title (or descriptor):	Cognitive Science
Commands to:	`listserv@nic.sufnet.nl`
Subscribe:	`subscribe COGSCI Your-name`
Unsubscribe:	`unsubscribe COGSCI`
List:	`COGSCI@nic.sufnet.nl`
List owner:	Michel Weenink (E-mail: `weenink@psych.kun.nl`)

This list is an open, unmoderated discussion about all aspects of cognitive science. Topics may include artificial intelligence, linguistics, philosophy, connectionism, psychology, conferences, lectures, and publications.

Title (or descriptor):	Community Psychology
Commands to:	listserv@maelstrom.stjohns.edu
Subscribe:	subscribe commpsy Your-name
Unsubscribe:	unsubscribe commpsy
List:	commpsy@maelstrom.stjohns.edu
List owners:	Bob Dick (E-mail: bdick@scu.edu.au)

This moderated list is for the discussion of community psychology. Community psychology as a field is devoted to helping psychologists understand and improve communities in ways that are helpful, cooperative, and culturally appropriate.

Title (or descriptor):	Computers in Mental Health
Web site:	http://groups.yahoo.com/group/CIMH2000/
Subscribe:	CIMH2000-subscribe@yahoogroups.com
Unsubscribe:	CIMH2000-unsubscribe@yahoogroups.com
List:	CIMH2000@yahoogroups.com
List owner(s):	Martin Briscoe (E-mail: M.H.Briscoe@exeter.ac.uk)
	Carl Littlejohns (E-mail: csljohns@cix.compulink.co.uk)

A closed list primarily for professionals interested in computer and software applications in the field of mental health. Topics discussed include billing and management software, assessment and treatment programs, information technology and its impact on the mental health field, ethics and confidentiality.

Title (or descriptor):	Counselors
Web site:	http://groups.yahoo.com/group/counselors/
Subscribe:	counselors-subscribe@yahoogroups.com
Unsubscribe:	counselors-unsubscribe@yahoogroups.com
List:	counselors@yahoogroups.com
List owner:	Edward S. Beck (E-mail: SusqInst@aol.com)

This professional forum is for behavioral health professionals to share and "dialogue outside the box." The mailing list includes psychiatrists, psychologists, marriage and family therapists, school counselors, mental health counselors, social workers, creative arts therapists, and other mental health professionals. The list is informal and active, allowing for frank, lively discussions on a wide range of topics.

Title (or descriptor):	Creative Arts Group Psychotherapy
Commands to:	`majordomo@albie.wcupa.edu`
Subscribe:	`subscribe grouptalk`
Unsubscribe:	`unsubscribe grouptalk`
List:	`grouptalk@albie.wcupa.edu`
List owner:	Tom Treadwell
	(E-mail: `ttreadwell@albie.wcupa.edu`)

This list offers discussion of all types of creative arts group psychotherapy among professionals—for instance, psychodrama and group psychotherapy—among other relevant and related topics.

Title (or descriptor):	Current Issues in Psychology and Psychiatry
Commands to:	`listserv@maelstrom.stjohns.edu`
Subscribe:	`subscribe PSYCH-CI Your-name`
Unsubscribe:	`unsubscribe PSYCH-CI`
List:	`PSYCH-CI@maelstrom.stjohns.edu`
List owner:	Ian Pitchford (E-mail: `I_Pitchford@msn.com`)

For the general discussion of topical issues in research and clinical practice in psychology, psychiatry, and related fields.

Title (or descriptor):	Disabilities, Social & Relational Context
Commands to:	`listserv@maelstrom.stjohns.edu`
Subscribe:	`subscribe disabled Your-name`
Unsubscribe:	`unsubscribe disabled`
List:	`disabled@maelstrom.stjohns.edu`

List owner(s):	D. S. Marks (E-mail: `d.s.marks@sheffield.ac.uk`)
	Ian Pitchford (E-mail: `I_Pitchford@msn.com`)

This list focuses on examining disability within a social and relational context. A dialectical approach to the body and psyche is emphasized.

Title (or descriptor):	Disaster Mental Health
Commands to:	`listserv@maelstrom.stjohns.edu`
Subscribe:	`subscribe DISASTMH Your-name`
Unsubscribe:	`unsubscribe DISASTMH`
List:	`DISASTMH@maelstrom.stjohns.edu`
List owner:	Denruth Lougeay (E-mail: `deneelou@cox.net`)

A forum for mental health professionals who work in the disaster and crisis fields.

Title (or descriptor):	Dissociative Disorders
Commands to:	`listserv@maelstrom.stjohns.edu`
Subscribe:	
	`subscribe dissociative-disorders Your-name`
Unsubscribe:	`unsubscribe dissociative-disorders`
List:	
	`dissociative-disorders@maelstrom.stjohns.edu`
List owner:	Peter Barach (E-mail: `pbarach@sprynet.com`)

This list offers discussion related to the diagnosis and treatment of dissociative disorders, including legal, theoretical, clinical, and ethical issues. This is a closed list for mental health professionals and graduate students only.

Title (or descriptor):	Dual-Diagnosis
Web site:	`http://users.erols.com/ksciacca`
Commands to:	`listserv@maelstrom.stjohns.edu`
Subscribe:	`subscribe dualdiag Your-name`
Unsubscribe:	`unsubscribe dualdiag`

List: `dualdiag@maelstrom.stjohns.edu`

List owner: Kathleen Sciacca (E-mail: `ksciacca@erols.com`)

This is a mailing list for co-occurring mental illness and substance disorders. Discussion regarding the theory, practice, treatment, research, and improved services for persons who have dual disorders is invited. This is a closed list for professionals only.

Title (or descriptor): Eating Disorders

Commands to: `listserv@maelstrom.stjohns.edu`

Subscribe: `subscribe eating-disorders Your-name`

Unsubscribe: `unsubscribe eating-disorders`

List: `eating-disorders@maelstrom.stjohns.edu`

List owner: David H. Gleaves (E-mail: `dhg@psyc.tamu.edu`)

This list is for the discussion of causes, treatment, theory, and research of eating disorders such as bulimia nervosa, obesity, and anorexia. Clinicians and researchers are welcomed.

Title (or descriptor): Evolutionary Approach to Human Development

Commands to: `listserv@maelstrom.stjohns.edu`

Subscribe: `subscribe sociobio Your-name`

Unsubscribe: `unsubscribe sociobio`

List: `sociobio@maelstrom.stjohns.edu`

List owner: F. Leon Wilson (E-mail: `flwilson@infinet.com`)

A professional discussion forum focused on the evolutionary approach to human development. It is intended to act as a resource for professionals and researchers interested in the fields of human ethology and sociobiology.

Title (or descriptor): Feminist Psychology

Web site:

`http://groups.yahoo.com/group/feminist-psychology/`

Subscribe:

feminist-psychology-subscribe@yahoogroups.com

Unsubscribe:

feminist-psychology-unsubscribe@yahoogroups.com

List: feminist-psychology@yahoogroups.com

A discussion group that explores women's and gender issues in psychology within a feminist framework.

Title (or descriptor):   Forensic Psychiatry/Psychology

Commands to: listserv@maelstrom.stjohns.edu

Subscribe: subscribe forensic-psych Your-name

Unsubscribe: unsubscribe forensic-psych

List: forensic-psych@maelstrom.stjohns.edu

List owner: Ron Schlensky (E-mail: rsmdjdl@aol.com)

Discussion of criminal and civil forensic psychiatry/psychology, including treatment issues, trial issues, disability insurance, and ethics.

Title (or descriptor):   Gestalt Theory

Web site:

http://groups.yahoo.com/group/gestalttheoryforum/

Subscribe:

gestalttheoryforum-subscribe@yahoogroups.com

Unsubscribe:

gestalttheoryforum-unsubscribe@yahoogroups.com

List: gestalttheoryforum@yahoogroups.com

This forum discusses Gestalt theory—as advocated by the likes of Wertheimer, Kohler, Koffka, and Lewin—and its application in psychology, psychotherapy, and related fields. This group is connected to the International Society for Gestalt Theory and Its Applications (http://www.enabling.org/ia/gestalt/ gerhards/).

Title (or descriptor):	Grants and Foundation Resources
Web site:	`http://charitychannel.com/forums/`
Commands to:	`listserv@philanthropy-review.com`
Subscribe:	`subscribe grants Your-name`
Unsubscribe:	`unsubscribe grants`
List:	`grants@philanthropy-review.com`

A forum that focuses on all aspects of grants and foundations.

Title (or descriptor):	Grants in Substance Abuse and Gun Violence
Web site:	

`http://www.jointogether.org/about/web/jtodirect/`

An announcement-only mailing list with national news, research, and alerts, and funding news and grant announcements for topics related to gun violence and substance abuse.

Title (or descriptor):	Group Psychotherapy
Commands to:	`listserv@lists.apa.org`
Subscribe:	`subscribe group-psychotherapy`
Unsubscribe:	`unsubscribe group-psychotherapy`
List:	`group-psychotherapy@lists.apa.org`
List owner:	Haim Weinberg (E-mail: `haimw@netvision.net.il`)

For any clinician who works with a group psychotherapeutic modality and for the discussion of group work and group psychotherapy.

Title (or descriptor):	Human Relations, Authority, and Justice
Commands to:	`listserv@maelstrom.stjohns.edu`
Subscribe:	`subscribe HRAJ Your-name`
Unsubscribe:	`unsubscribe HRAJ`
List:	`HRAJ@maelstrom.stjohns.edu`

List owners:	Robert Young (E-mail: `robert@rmy1.demon.co.uk`)
	Ian Pitchford (E-mail: `I_Pitchford@msn.com`)

Designed to encourage the application of psychoanalytic and related psychody-namic approaches to the understanding of group, institutional, cultural, and political processes.

Title (or descriptor):	Human Resources Network (HRNET)
Web site:	`http://groups.yahoo.com/group/HRNET/`
Subscribe:	`HRNET-subscribe@yahoogroups.com`
Unsubscribe:	`HRNET-unsubscribe@yahoogroups.com`
List:	`HRNET@yahoogroups.com`

This active forum is for professionals interested in research and the practice of human resource management. Topics include research ideas, statistical methods, research measures, teaching methods, and sharing resources and new research articles in the field.

Title (or descriptor):	Human Rights in Psychiatry (Dendrite)
Web site:	
	`http://mailman.efn.org/cgi-bin/listinfo/dendrite`
List:	`dendrite@efn.org`
List owner:	David Oaks (E-mail: `dendron@efn.org`)

This resource is a one-way mailing list, which sends periodic announcements (about twice a month) to list members about human rights in—and alternatives to—psychiatry. A service of Support Coalition's Web site.

Title (or descriptor):	Human Service Information Technology Applications
Web site:	`http://www.husita.org/`
Commands to:	`listserv@listserv.uta.edu`
Subscribe:	`subscribe husita Your-name`
Unsubscribe:	`unsubscribe husita`

List:	hsuita@listserv.uta.edu
List owner:	Dick Schoech (E-mail: schoech@uta.edu)

This forum is for the professional discussion of the application of information technology and information management in human services.

Title (or descriptor):	Hypnosis
Commands to:	listserv@maelstrom.stjohns.edu
Subscribe:	subscribe hypnosis Your-name
Unsubscribe:	unsubscribe hypnosis
List:	hypnosis@maelstrom.stjohns.edu
List owner:	Irving Kirsch (E-mail: IRVINGK@uconnvm.uconn.edu)

This forum is for the discussion of hypnosis and the broader topics of suggestion and suggestibility. It is a closed list, open to researchers and scientifically minded clinicians who would like to exchange ideas and information on these topics.

Title (or descriptor):	Industrial and Organizational Psychology (IOOB-L)
Commands to:	listserv@uga.cc.uga.edu
Subscribe:	subscribe IOOB-L Your-name
Unsubscribe:	unsubscribe IOOB-L
List:	IOOB-L@uga.cc.uga.edu
List owner:	John L. Cofer (E-mail: coferjl@utk.edu)

A discussion list dedicated to industrial/organizational psychology and organization behavior (IOOB).

Title (or descriptor):	Informatics Review Newsletter
Web site:	
	http://www.topica.com/lists/Informatics-Review/
Subscribe:	Informatics-Review-subscribe@topica.com
Unsubscribe:	Informatics-Review-subscribe@topica.com
List:	Informatics-Review-subscribe@topica.com

The Informatics Review Newsletter is an announcement-only mailing list that is intended to help clinicians and information technology professionals keep current with the latest developments in the field of clinical computing (a subfield of medical informatics). Sponsored by *The Informatics Review* (`http://www.informatics-review.com/`).

Title (or descriptor):	International Society for Mental Health Online
Web site:	`http://www.ismho.org/`
Subscribe:	`ismho-general-subscribe@yahoogroups.com`
Unsubscribe:	`ismho-general-unsubscribe@yahoogroups.com`
List:	`ismho-general@yahoogroups.com`

The open discussion forum for the International Society for Mental Health Online, an organization formed in 1997 to promote the understanding, use, and development of online communication, information, and technology for the international mental health community.

Title (or descriptor):	Internships, Psychology
Commands to:	`listserv@listserv.utk.edu`
Subscribe:	`subscribe INTERN-L Your-name`
Unsubscribe:	`unsubscribe INTERN-L`
List:	`intern-L@listserv.utk.edu`
List owner:	Victor W. Barr (E-mail: `ybarr@.utk.edu`)

This forum is designed to foster discussion of the psychology internship process and is open to all current and prospective interns, as well as internship program staff.

Title (or descriptor):	Joint Commission Accreditation
Web site:	

`http://lyris.ucg.com/cgi-bin/lyris.pl?enter=jcaho-watch`

For discussions on the process of obtaining Joint Commission Accreditation.

Title (or descriptor):	Latin Psych
Commands to:	`listserv@maelstrom.stjohns.edu`
Subscribe:	`subscribe lat-psy Your-name`
Unsubscribe:	`unsubscribe lat-psy`
List:	`lat-psy@maelstrom.stjohns.edu`
List owner:	Hector R. Biaggi (E-mail: `biaggi@bellsouth.net`)

This list is to encourage communication among Latin mental health professionals around the world. Its main languages are Spanish, Portuguese, and English, in that order. It has a significant South American representation and a strong clinical orientation.

Title (or descriptor):	Learned Helplessness
Web site:	
	`http://www.psych.upenn.edu/~fresco/helplessness.html`
Commands to:	`listserv@lists.apa.org`
Subscribe:	`subscribe helplessness`
Unsubscribe:	`unsubscribe helplessness`
List:	`helplessness@lists.apa.org`
List owners:	David Fresco
	(E-mail: `fresco@cattell.psych.upenn.edu`)

This forum is for the discussion of research on learned helplessness and explanatory style. Topics may include biological substratum, depression, anxiety, preventions, CAVE, politics, children, personal control, health, battering, bereavement, PTSD, sex differences, pessimism, work, and heritability issues.

Title (or descriptor):	Learning—Behavior, Models, Theory
Commands to:	`listserv@maelstrom.stjohns.edu`
Subscribe:	`subscribe learning Your-name`
Unsubscribe:	`unsubscribe learning`
List:	`learning@maelstrom.stjohns.edu`
List owner:	Garry A. Flint
	(E-mail: `gaflint@emotional-freedom.com`)

This list is for the discussion of human behavioral and experiential phenomena and developing models of learning. It is opened to researchers and clinicians interested in a discussion of learning models of human behavior or experiential phenomenon.

Title (or descriptor):	Managed Behavioral Healthcare
Commands to:	`listserv@maelstrom.stjohns.edu`
Subscribe:	`subscribe MBHC Your-name`
Unsubscribe:	`unsubscribe MBHC`
List:	`MBHC@maelstrom.stjohns.edu`
List owners:	Greg Alter (E-mail: `alter@surf.com`)
	Deborah Teplow (E-mail: `debtep@ix.netcom.com`)

This list is for the discussion of the managed behavioral health care field. Topics may include health care reform, best clinical practices, insurance benefits, group practice structures, outcome research, and informatics.

Title (or descriptor):	Marriage and Family Therapy Counseling
Commands to:	`listserv@maelstrom.stjohns.edu`
Subscribe:	`subscribe MFTC-L Your-name`
Unsubscribe:	`unsubscribe MFTC-L`
List:	`MFTC-L@maelstrom.stjohns.edu`
List owners:	Leonard Bohanon (E-mail: `boha@hal-pc.org`) and
	Richard Sies (E-mail: `rsies@dmci.net`)

This group is for the discussion of issues related to marriage and family therapy and areas of interest to marriage and family therapists. Although opinions from varied theoretical approaches are encouraged, the discussions are often narrative and solution focused.

Title (or descriptor):   Medical Informatics

Web site:

    `http://groups.yahoo.com/group/medicalinformatics/`

Subscribe:

    `medicalinformatics-subscribe@yahoogroups.com`

Unsubscribe:

`medicalinformatics-unsubscribe@yahoogroups.com`

List: `medicalinformatics@yahoogroups.com`

A forum devoted to image processing, computerized patient records, decision support systems, telemedicine topics, and Web-based solutions in medical and health care practice.

Title (or descriptor):   Mental Health in the Media

Commands to: `listserv@lists.apa.org`

Subscribe: `subscribe PSY-MEDIA`

Unsubscribe: `unsubscribe PSY-MEDIA`

List: `PSY-MEDIA@lists.apa.org`

List owner: Les Posen (E-mail: `lesposen@enternet.com.au`)

Features a broad discussion of public perception and portrayal of mental health and mental health issues.

Title (or descriptor):   Mental Health Workers

Commands to: `listserv@maelstrom.stjohns.edu`

Subscribe: `subscribe MENTAL-HEALTH-WORKER Your-name`

Unsubscribe: `unsubscribe MENTAL-HEALTH-WORKER`

List:

`mental-health-worker@maelstrom.stjohns.edu`

List owner: George Blake
                             (E-mail: `mental-health-worker-info@aapt.com`)

This forum is for individuals interested in, working in, or supervising those in entry-level psychology, psychiatry, and mental health jobs requiring a bachelors degree or less.

Title (or descriptor):   Net Dynamics

Web site: `http://www.enabling.org/ia/netdynam/`

Commands to: `listserv@maelstrom.stjohns.edu`

Subscribe:	`subscribe netdynam Your-name`
Unsubscribe:	`unsubscribe netdynam`
List:	`netdynam@maelstrom.stjohns.edu`
List owner:	O. Simon Onken (E-mail: `simon@loris.net`)

This list examines online group dynamics, covering topics such as the perceptions of the other list participants, the dynamics of flame wars, power and persuasion, and what is effective communication and why.

Title (or descriptor): Pastoral Counseling

Web site:

    `http://groups.yahoo.com/group/pastoral-counseling/`

Subscribe:

    `pastoral-counseling-subscribe@yahoogroups.com`

Unsubscribe:

    `pastoral-counseling-unsubscribe@yahoogroups.com`

List: `pastoral-counseling@yahoogroups.com`

This multifaith forum comprises mainly members of the Association of Pastoral Counselors (`http://www.aapc.org/`) discussing issues related to the field of pastoral counseling. Professionals in pastoral counseling have experience and backgrounds in theology as well as counseling. This group allows members to discuss issues such as the integration of psychotherapy and spirituality in many faith traditions, exchange news and resources, and network with other pastoral counselors.

Title (or descriptor):	Philopsychy Society
Commands to:	`majordomo@listserver.hkbu.edu.hk`
Subscribe:	`subscribe PPS-L`
Unsubscribe:	`unsubscribe PPS-L`
List:	`PPS-L@listserver.hkbu.edu.hk`
List owner:	Stephen Palmquist (E-mail: `stevepq@hkbu.edu.hk`)

This serves as a forum for discussing issues of interest to members of the Philopsychy Society. Topics may include the interface between philosophy and psychology, any philosophical or psychological topics that are likely to enhance our understanding of the theory and practice of "soul-loving" ("philopsychy"), topics from any area of academia (or life in general) that are likely to accomplish the latter goal.

Title (or descriptor):	Political Science–Psychology/Psychiatry
Commands to:	`listserv@maelstrom.stjohns.edu`
Subscribe:	`subscribe POLI-PSY Your-name`
Unsubscribe:	`unsubscribe POLI-PSY`
List:	`POLI-PSY@maelstrom.stjohns.edu`
List owner:	George Blake (E-mail: `poli-psy-info@aapt.com`)

A forum for the discussion of the politics and political aspects, theories, and research of psychology and psychiatry.

Title (or descriptor):	Postmodern Therapies
Commands to:	`listserv@maelstrom.stjohns.edu`
Subscribe:	`subscribe PMTH Your-name`
Unsubscribe:	`unsubscribe PMTH`
List:	`PMTH@maelstrom.stjohns.edu`
List owner:	Lois Shawver (E-mail: `rathbone@california.com`)

This forum is for licensed therapists, graduate student therapists, and scholars or academics interested in the topic of psychotherapy. The group focuses on a collaborative discussion of psychotherapy theory. The list is "postmodern" in that most subscribers are suspicious of metanarratives in psychotherapy theory.

Title (or descriptor):	Psybernet
Web site:	`http://groups.yahoo.com/group/psyber-l/`
Subscribe:	`psyber-l-subscribe@yahoogroups.com`
Unsubscribe:	`psyber-l-unsubscribe@yahoogroups.com`
List:	`psyber-l@yahoogroups.com`
List owner:	Walter Logeman (E-mail: `walter@psybernet.co.nz`)

This is a forum devoted to the experiential exploration of the psyche in cyberspace. Topics may include leadership skills in the administration of mailing lists, list dynamics, depth psychology on the Internet, and professional services on the Internet.

Title (or descriptor):	Psychiatric Epidemiology
Commands to:	`listserv@maelstrom.stjohns.edu`
Subscribe:	`subscribe PSYCHEPI Your-name`
Unsubscribe:	`unsubscribe PSYCHEPI`
List:	`PSYCHEPI@maelstrom.stjohns.edu`
List owner:	George Blake (E-mail: `psychepi-info@aapt.com`)

A group focused on the professional discussion of the quantitative study of the distribution and causes of mental disorders in human populations. The goal is to add to knowledge concerning etiology, natural history, treatment and prevention of psychiatric disorders. Topics include case identification, genetic/family studies, recurrence and comorbidity, social functioning, treatment efficacy, iatrogenic effects, and health care delivery systems.

Title (or descriptor):	Psychiatric Nursing
Web site:	

`http://www.jiscmail.ac.uk/lists/psychiatric-nursing`
`.html`

Commands to:	`listserv@jiscmail.ac.uk`
Subscribe:	`subscribe psychiatric-nursing your-name`
Unsubscribe:	`unsubscribe psychiatric-nursing`
List:	`psychiatric-nursing@jiscmail.ac.uk`
List owners:	Len Bowers (E-mail: `l.bowers@city.ac.uk`)

For the discussion of issues facing psychiatric nurses, centering around clinical practice topics.

Title (or descriptor):	Psychiatric Social Workers
Commands to:	`listserv@maelstrom.stjohns.edu`
Subscribe:	`subscribe PSYC-SOC Your-name`
Unsubscribe:	`unsubscribe PSYC-SOC`
List:	`PSYC-SOC@maelstrom.stjohns.edu`

List owner:	Beverly Jamison (E-mail: `bjamison@marymount.edu`)

For the discussion of issues of interest to psychiatric social workers.

Title (or descriptor):	Psychiatry
Commands to:	`listserv@maelstrom.stjohns.edu`
Subscribe:	`subscribe PSYCHL Your-name`
Unsubscribe:	`unsubscribe PSYCHL`
List:	`PSYCHL@maelstrom.stjohns.edu`
List owner:	Beverly Jamison (E-mail: `bjamison@marymount.edu`)

This is a list primarily for mental health professionals to discuss theories of psychopathology, methods for critical assessment of theories and practices, relevant research with emphasis on the interrelationship of theory, fact, and practice. This list also encourages the exchange of views on research and theory regarding psychopathology with particular emphasis on application to practice of all sorts.

Title (or descriptor):   PsychLawExperts

Web site:

`http://groups.yahoo.com/group/PsychLawExperts/`

Subscribe:

`PsychLawExperts-subscribe@yahoogroups.com`

Unsubscribe:

`PsychLawExperts-unsubscribe@yahoogroups.com`

List: `PsychLawExperts@yahoogroups.com`

For discussion of all areas relating to psychology/psychiatry and the law, including political, social, and economic issues and civil rights and civil liberties concerns.

Title (or descriptor):	Psychoanalysis
Commands to:	`listserv@maelstrom.stjohns.edu`

Subscribe:	subscribe psychoan Your-name
Unsubscribe:	unsubscribe psychoan
List:	psychoan@maelstrom.stjohns.edu
List owner:	Robert Galatzer-Levy
	(E-mail: gala@midway.uchicago.edu)

A forum to host issues of psychoanalytic practice, theory, politics, history, and the application of psychoanalysis to other disciplines.

Title (or descriptor):   Psychoanalysis and Psychotherapy

Web site:

http://groups.yahoo.com/group/psychoanalysis-and-psychotherapy/

Subscribe:

psychoanalysis-and-psychotherapy-subscribe@yahoogroups.com

Unsubscribe:

psychoanalysis-and-psychotherapy-unsubscribe@yahoogroups.com

List:

psychoanalysis-and-psychotherapy@yahoogroups.com

A forum for all individuals interested in the psychoanalytic approach as employed in analysis, psychoanalytic psychotherapy and psychodynamic counseling. This group is meant to foster communication across those three communities, both in theory and in practice.

Title (or descriptor):	Psychoanalysis and the Public Sphere
Commands to:	listproc@sheffield.ac.uk
Subscribe:	subscribe psa-public-sphere Your-name
Unsubscribe:	unsubscribe psa-public-sphere
List:	psa-public-sphere@sheffield.ac.uk
List owners:	Robert Young (E-mail: robert@rmy1.demon.co.uk) and Mark Alexander
	(E-mail: m.alexander@wellcome.ac.uk)

For discussion of wider social, cultural, political, ideological, institutional, and related aspects of psychoanalysis and other psychodynamic approaches.

Title (or descriptor):   Psychoanalytic Studies

Web site:

`http://www.shef.ac.uk/uni/academic/N-Q/psysc/`
`psastud.html`

Commands to: `listproc@sheffield.ac.uk`

Subscribe: `subscribe psychoanalytic-studies`
`Your-name`

Unsubscribe: `unsubscribe psychoanalytic-studies`

List: `psychoanalytic-studies@sheffield.ac.uk`

List owners: Sean Homer (E-mail: `s.i.homer@sheffield,ac.uk`)
and Tim Kendall
(E-mail: `t.j.kendall@sheffield.ac.uk`)

For scholarly discussion of psychoanalysis and related psychodynamic approaches; topics may include anything that has a psychoanalytic or psychodynamic dimension.

Title (or descriptor):   Psychodrama

Commands to: `listserv@maelstrom.stjohns.edu`

Subscribe: `subscribe psychodrama Your-name`

Unsubscribe: `unsubscribe psychodrama`

List: `psychodrama@maelstrom.stjohns.edu`

List owner: Danilo Curci (E-mail: `quadrant@iol.it`)

A forum to discuss, act, and develop old and new ideas, projects, suggestions on Moreno's psychodrama, role-playing, cathartic narration, and other kinds of educational and therapeutical dramalike interaction.

Title (or descriptor):   Psychologists, Clinical

Commands to: `listserv@listserv.nodak.edu`

Subscribe:

`subscribe clinical-psychologists Your-name`

Unsubscribe:	`unsubscribe clinical-psychologists`
List:	
	`clinical-psychologists@listserv.nodak.edu`
List owner:	Joseph Plaud (E-mail: `plaud@fdrheritage.org`)

This forum is the central online discussion area for clinical psychologists to congregate and share ideas that occupy the broad area of clinical psychology. Clinical case conferences are welcomed, as are discussion on treatment and research within clinical psychology and closely related areas.

Title (or descriptor):	Psychologists, Division 12 of APA
Commands to:	`listserv@listserv.nodak.edu`
Subscribe:	`subscribe DIV12 Your-name`
Unsubscribe:	`unsubscribe DIV12`
List:	`DIV12@listserv.nodak.edu`
List owner:	Joseph Plaud (E-mail: `plaud@fdrheritage.org`)

This is the official mailing list for members of Division 12 (Clinical Psychology) of the American Psychological Association. Its primary function is to serve as a means of communication and rapid dissemination of knowledge on issues ranging from the governance of clinical psychology to research and clinical issues relating to the science and practice of clinical psychology.

Title (or descriptor):	Psychologists, National List (PsyUSA)
Commands to:	`listserv@maelstrom.stjohns.edu`
Subscribe:	`subscribe PsyUSA Your-name`
Unsubscribe:	`unsubscribe PsyUSA`
List:	`PsyUSA@maelstrom.stjohns.edu`

This long-standing and popular list was formed to network practicing psychologists. Topics include the dissemination of announcements on practice management, treatment resources, insurance companies and HMOs, job openings, computer software (clinical, office, and billing), new practice opportunities and sale of practices, legal and liability issues, requests for consultations, referrals, treatment protocols and guidelines, business methods, practice economics, advanced training and certifications, federal and state legislation affecting psychology, issues of various psychological associations, and changes and trends in behavioral health care delivery structures. Contact the list owner for additional information about the entire PsyUSA network, which consists of individual state mailing lists and two additional national lists (see below) for discussion of the latest news, trends, information, and opinions permeating the mental health care field. This list can get very busy at times.

Title (or descriptor):	Psychologists, National List (PsyChat)
Commands to:	`listserv@maelstrom.stjohns.edu`
Subscribe:	`subscribe PsyChat Your-name`
Unsubscribe:	`unsubscribe PsyChat`
List:	`PsyChat@maelstrom.stjohns.edu`

A part of the PsyUSA Network of associated mailing lists, this national list encourages informal group conversations among psychologists, light-hearted dialogue, "opportunities to develop personal relationships with other [. . .] subscribers, and other kinds of comradery" (from the public description of this list).

Title (or descriptor):	Psychologists, National List (PsyPOV)
Commands to:	`listserv@maelstrom.stjohns.edu`
Subscribe:	`subscribe PsyPOV Your-name`
Unsubscribe:	`unsubscribe PsyPOV`
List:	`PsyPOV@maelstrom.stjohns.edu`

PsyPOV (Point of View) is a part of the PsyUSA Network of associated mailing lists. This national list encourages debate among psychologists on various topical and timely issues, such as managed care, ethics, psychotherapy treatment, training issues, supervision, etc.

Title (or descriptor):	Psychologists, Practice
Commands to:	`listserv@lists.apa.org`
Subscribe:	`subscribe practice Your-name`
Unsubscribe:	`unsubscribe practice`
List:	`practice@lists.apa.org`

For psychologist members of the American Psychological Association to discuss practice issues.

Title (or descriptor):	Psychology and Technology
Commands to:	listserv@maelstrom.stjohns.edu
Subscribe:	subscribe PsyTech
Unsubscribe:	unsubscribe PsyTech Your-name
List:	PsyTech@maelstrom.stjohns.edu

This forum is devoted to aiding the propagation of new technology in psychological practice, research, and teaching. It is a member of the PsyUSA Network of associated mailing lists.

Title (or descriptor):	Psychology in Behavioral Health Practice
Commands to:	listserv@maelstrom.stjohns.edu
Subscribe:	subscribe psymed Your-name
Unsubscribe:	unsubscribe psymed
List:	psymed@maelstrom.stjohns.edu

A forum for the discussion of assessment techniques and treatment methods applicable to behavioral health problems, the application of psychology to lifestyle and behavior changes in the prevention of health problems, employment opportunities in behavioral health, maintianing relationships with physicians and other health care providers, and sources of information accessible via the Internet that are relevant to behavioral health.

Title (or descriptor):	Psychology, Developmental Disabilities
Commands to:	listserv@listserv.nodak.edu
Subscribe:	subscribe PSYCH-DD Your-name
Unsubscribe:	unsubscribe PSYCH-DD
List:	PSYCH-DD@listserv.nodak.edu
List owner:	Paul Kolstoe (E-mail: pdkolstoe@yahoo.com)

The purpose of this list is to promote professional discussion of psychological issues of people with developmental disabilities.

Title (or descriptor):   Psychology Graduate Students

Commands to: `listserv@lists.apa.org`

Subscribe: `subscribe PSYCGRAD Your-name`

Unsubscribe: `unsubscribe PSYCGRAD`

List: `psycgrad@lists.apa.org`

A vehicle for graduate students in psychology to communicate ideas and share information about conferences worldwide.

Title (or descriptor):   Psychology in Law Enforcement

Commands to: `listserv@maelstrom.stjohns.edu`

Subscribe: `subscribe psycop Your-name`

Unsubscribe: `unsubscribe psycop`

List: `psycop@maelstrom.stjohns.edu`

A discussion list for police psychologists on the delivery of psychological services to law enforcement personnel.

Title (or descriptor):   Psychology of Women

Commands to: `listerv@pete.uri.edu`

Subscribe: `subscribe POWR-L Your-name`

Unsubscribe: `unsubscribe POWR-L`

List: `POWR-L@pete.uri.edu`

The purpose of this forum is to facilitate discussion of current topics, research, teaching strategies, and practice issues among people interested in the discipline of psychology of women, and to publicize relevant conferences, job announcements, calls for papers, publications, and the like. It is open to anyone interested in the field.

Title (or descriptor):   Psychology of Women, International

Subscribe: E-mail Irene Hanson Frieze at `frieze@pitt.edu`

This group is for feminist psychologists interested in international issues.

Title (or descriptor):	Psychometrics
Web site:	http://groups.yahoo.com/group/Psychometrics/
Subscribe:	Psychometrics-subscribe@yahoogroups.com
Unsubscribe:	

Psychometrics-unsubscribe@yahoogroups.com

List:	Psychometrics@yahoogroups.com

This discussion group is aimed at psychometric test developers, researchers, and students who want to discuss approaches to test development, reliability assessment, and validation.

Title (or descriptor):	Psychotherapists in Training
Commands to:	listserv@maelstrom.stjohns.edu
Subscribe:	subscribe PIT-D Your-name
Unsubscribe:	unsubscribe PIT-D
List:	PIT-D@maelstrom.stjohns.edu
List owners:	Jessica Percodani (E-mail: Jessica-Percodani@worldnet.att.net)

A list for all psychotherapists in training—at all levels of training—for the discussion of training issues, supervisory relationships, and therapy experiences.

Title (or descriptor):	Psychotherapy, European
Web site:	http://groups.yahoo.com/group/europsych/
Subscribe:	europsych-subscribe@yahoogroups.com
Unsubscribe:	europsych-unsubscribe@yahoogroups.com
List:	europsych@yahoogroups.com
List owner:	Robert M. Young (E-mail: robert@rmy1.demon.co.uk)

This forum was created to help foster the exchange of information about psychotherapy in all of Europe. Information about psychotherapy facilities, as well as training and research in various European countries is shared. Practitioners of all approaches of psychotherapy are welcomed.

Title (or descriptor): Psychotherapy and Spirituality

Web site:

`http://groups.yahoo.com/group/Psychotherapy-and-Spirituality/`

Subscribe:

`Psychotherapy-and-Spirituality-subscribe@yahoogroups.com`

Unsubscribe:

`Psychotherapy-and-Spirituality-unsubscribe@yahoogroups.com`

List:

`Psychotherapy-and-Spirituality@yahoogroups.com`

A group for sharing insights and experiences related to psychotherapy, spirituality, and the interconnections between the two. Topics include religions such as Buddhism, Taoism, Islam, Christianity, Hinduism, Judaism; mental health, psychotic episodes, depressions, schizophrenia; spiritual emergency; Kundalini; chacra; process work, Gestalt therapy, Hakomi therapy; meditation, prayer; psychosynthesis; transpersonal therapy; primal therapy; yoga; and shamanism, among others.

Title (or descriptor): Psychotherapy Networker

Web site: `http://www.topica.com/lists/ftnetwork/`

Subscribe: `ftnetwork-subscribe@topica.com`

Unsubscribe: `ftnetwork-unsubscribe@topica.com`

List: `ftnetwork@topica.com`

This is a broad forum for professional discussions on issues, trends, research, workshops, and other ideas that affect the emotional health of individuals, couples, families, and their communities. List members also share referrals and ideas for improving clinical skills and expanding practices. Sponsored by the *Psychotherapy Networker* magazine (`http://www.psychotherapynetworker.com/`).

Title (or descriptor): Psychotherapy–Pharmacotherapy Comparative Outcome Research

Commands to: `listserv@maelstrom.stjohns.edu`

Subscribe: `subscribe PSY-PHAR Your-name`

Unsubscribe: `unsubscribe PSY-PHAR`

List: `PSY-PHAR@maelstrom.stjohns.edu`

List owner: Pete Watts (E-mail: `awatt04@students.bbk.ac.uk`)

This is a forum for psychologists, psychiatrists, and other mental health researchers and clinicians to discuss topics regarding psychotherapy–pharmacotherapy comparative outcome research. Empirical, theoretical, and case-based discussions are welcomed.

Title (or descriptor): REBT-Cognitive Behavioral Therapy

Web site:

   `http://groups.yahoo.com/group/REBT-CBT-FORUM/`

Subscribe:

   `REBT-CBT-FORUM-subscribe@yahoogroups.com`

Unsubscribe:

   `REBT-CBT-FORUM-unsubscribe@yahoogroups.com`

List: `REBT-CBT-FORUM@yahoogroups.com`

A forum for professionals and lay persons to discuss rational emotive behavior therapy (REBT) and cognitive behavioral therapy. Other cognitive behavioral techniques, such as reality therapy, multimodal therapy, and schema therapy, are also welcomed.

Title (or descriptor): Research Design

Commands to: `listserv@lists.apa.org`

Subscribe: `subscribe research-design`

Unsubscribe: `unsubscribe research-design`

List: `research-design@lists.apa.org`

List owner: B. Hudnall Stamm (E-mail: `bhstamm@isu.edu`)

For researchers in the behavioral health sciences to discuss issues of research and study design and statistics.

Title (or descriptor):	Rorschach
Commands to:	listserv@maelstrom.stjohns.edu
Subscribe:	subscribe rorschach Your-name
Unsubscribe:	unsubscribe rorschach
List:	rorschach@maelstrom.stjohns.edu
List owner:	Jack Gerber (E-mail: jackgerber@comcast.net)

For the general discussion of the Rorschach Inkblot test.

Title (or descriptor):	Rural Care
Commands to:	listserv@lists.apa.org
Subscribe:	subscribe rural-care
Unsubscribe:	unsubscribe rural-care
List:	rural-care@lists.apa.org
List owner:	B. Hudnall Stamm (E-mail: bhstamm@isu.edu)

This list is for the support of health care workers isolated in rural and bush communities, and for the continuing dialogue of those concerned with health care delivery in remote and developing areas worldwide. The forum is intended for health care workers in all types of settings.

Title (or descriptor):	Self Relations Psychotherapy
Commands to:	listserv@maelstrom.stjohns.edu
Subscribe:	subscribe SR-L Your-name
Unsubscribe:	unsubscribe SR-L
List:	SR-L@maelstrom.stjohns.edu
List owner:	Leonard Bohanon (E-mail: Boha@hal-pc.org)

This forum is for individuals interested in self-relations psychotherapy. It is intended for practicing psychotherapists and graduate or professional students in mental health disciplines.

Title (or descriptor):   Sexual Disability Research
Web site:
    `http://groups.yahoo.com/group/SexDisabilityResearc/`
Subscribe:
    `SexDisabilityResearc-subscribe@yahoogroups.com`
Unsubscribe:
    `SexDisabilityResearc-unsubscribe@yahoogroups.com`
List: `SexDisabilityResearc@yahoogroups.com`

For the discussion of research issues relating to sexuality and disability.

Title (or descriptor):   Sleep Technology
Commands to: `listserv@dartmouth.edu`
Subscribe: `subscribe SLPTECH Your-name`
Unsubscribe: `unsubscribe SLPTECH`
List: `SLPTECH@dartmouth.edu`
List owner: Mary MacDonald
                               (E-mail: `Mary.M.MacDonald@dartmouth.edu`)

A moderated discussion forum for all issues regarding sleep technology.

Title (or descriptor):   Social Science Data Discussion
Commands to: `listproc@irss.unc.edu`
Subscribe: `subscribe SOS-DATA Your-name`
Unsubscribe: `unsubscribe SOS-DATA`
List: `SOS-DATA@irss.unc.edu`
List owner: Jim Cassell (E-mail: `irsslmgr@unc.edu`)

This is a forum for discussion of any topic related to social science data. Topics may include references to sources of data on some particular subject, conference announcements, new data sources, announcements of data archives, and information sources available online.

Title (or descriptor):	Social Work
Commands to:	listproc@lists.vcu.edu
Subscribe:	subscribe SCIOFSLW Your-name
Unsubscribe:	unsubscribe SCIOFSLW
List:	SCIOFSLW@lists.vcu.edu
List owner:	W. Beverly (E-mail: wbeverly@mail1.vcu.edu)

For the discussion of issues related to social work.

Title (or descriptor):	Social Work–Social Issues
Web site:	http://groups.yahoo.com/group/socialwork/
Subscribe:	socialwork-subscribe@yahoogroups.com
Unsubscribe:	socialwork-unsubscribe@yahoogroups.com
List:	socialwork@yahoogroups.com

This group is dedicated primarily to those persons interested in discussing current issues in social work.

Title (or descriptor):	Telehealth
Commands to:	listserv@maelstrom.stjohns.edu
Subscribe:	subscribe telehealth Your-name
Unsubscribe:	unsubscribe telehealth
List:	telehealth@maelstrom.stjohns.edu

A professional discussion list focused on telehealth ethics, laws, research, services, and technologies amongst mental health professionals.

Title (or descriptor):	Therapists in Recovery from Addiction
Commands to:	listserv@maelstrom.stjohns.edu

Subscribe:	`subscribe TREAD Your-name`
Unsubscribe:	`unsubscribe TREAD`
List:	`TREAD@maelstrom.stjohns.edu`

This is a closed mutual support list for therapists who are in recovery from addictions including alcoholism, substance addiction, and other "addictive" behaviors. The list membership is restricted to professional, licensed therapists, or therapists in professional training who consider themselves to be in recovery from an addiction.

Title (or descriptor):	Transformational Processing
Web site:	`http://www.worldtrans.org/transproc.html`
Commands to:	`majordomo@newciv.org`
Subscribe:	`subscribe TRANSPROC-L`
Unsubscribe:	`unsubscribe TRANSPROC-L`
List:	`TRANSPROC-L@newciv.org`
List owner:	Flemming Funch (E-mail: `ffunch@newciv.org`)

A forum for the serious student of the transformational processing system of personal counseling techniques developed by Flemming Funch.

Title (or descriptor):	Transcultural Psychology
Commands to:	`listserv@listserv.nodak.edu`
Subscribe:	

    subscribe transcultural-psychology Your-name

Unsubscribe:	`unsubscribe transcultural-psychology`
List:	

    transcultural-psychology@listserv.nodak.edu

List owners:	Sunkyo Kwon (E-mail: `kwon@tu-berlin.de`)

This forum is for the exchange of ideas, opinions, and information in cross-cultural research, minority issues, and "indigenous psychologies." Intended for mental health professionals and professionals-to-be in both academic and applied settings, participation of individuals in other disciplines is actively encouraged to add diversity and variety.

Title (or descriptor):	Traumatic Stress
Commands to:	`listserv@lists.apa.org`
Subscribe:	`subscribe traumatic-stress`
Unsubscribe:	`unsubscribe traumatic-stress`
List:	`traumatic-stress@lists.apa.org`
List owner:	Various (E-mail: `traumatic-stress-request@listp.apa.org`)

The purpose of this forum is to promote the investigation, assessment, and treatment of immediate and long-term psychosocial, physiological, and existential consequences of highly stressful (traumatic) events. Includes discussion of posttraumatic stress disorder.

Title (or descriptor):	Women's Studies
Commands to:	`listerv@umdd.umd.edu`
Subscribe:	`subscribe WMST-L Your-name`
Unsubscribe:	`unsubscribe WMST-L`
List:	`WMST-L@umdd.umd.edu`

This forum is for individuals involved in women's studies as teachers, researchers, librarians, and/or program administrators. Topics include current research, teaching strategies, useful texts and films, innovative courses, funding sources, building women's studies majors, minors, and graduate programs, relations between women's studies and other "minority studies" programs, and other academic issues.

Title (or descriptor):	Victim Assistance
Web site:	`http://www.vaonline.org/vaform.html`

The forum acts as an aid to increase communication between the many public, private, police, judicial, and governmental victim-assistance organizations that exist worldwide, as well as between individuals involved in this field. It also provides a place for support of professionals working in this area, announcements of related conferences and workshops, and a discussion forum for ideas and solutions to dealing with problems victims face.

Title (or descriptor):	Youth–Anxiety–Depression
Commands to:	listserv@maelstrom.stjohns.edu
Subscribe:	subscribe YANX-DEP Your-name
Unsubscribe:	unsubscribe YANX-DEP
List:	YANX-DEP@maelstrom.stjohns.edu
List owner:	Meg Smith (E-mail: m.smith@uws.edu.au)

Focused specifically on anxiety and depression amongst children and adolescents. The group is interdisciplinary and welcomes mental health professionals, in addition to parents and children affected by depression or anxiety. The forum takes an empirical approach to the nature, etiology, assessment, and treatment of anxiety and depression problems in children and adolescents.

Newsgroup Discussions

Newsgroups are the more public discussion forums available through the Internet. Their readerships typically number in the tens of thousands (compared to the few hundred on most mailing lists). In the psychology and mental health newsgroups, the readership consists largely of laypeople, not professionals. It is for these reasons that most professionals tend to stick to mailing lists, which give the appearance of more intimacy and confidentiality.

Newsgroups are accessed through software commonly provided as a part of your online account. Newsgroup software is often referred to as a "newsgroup reader," and one is built into the Netscape software. The procedure to subscribe to a newsgroup varies according to the type software you use, so there's no particular method I can describe here. Further information on how to subscribe to a new newsgroup or remove current subscriptions is available through the "Help" file in such software.

Nonetheless, newsgroups may provide a good forum for asking a general research or clinical question where a wide variety of opinions is desired. Some newsgroups are moderated, which tends to increase the quality of the discussion. The moderator ensures only those messages of relevance to the forum get posted. Table 6.1 offers a list of relevant professional newsgroups in alphabetical order by topic.

TABLE 6.1 Professional Newsgroups

Description	Newsgroup Name	Moderated?
Adler, Alfred	`alt.psychology.adlerian`	No
Announcements of interest to psychologists and mental health professionals in general	`sci.psychology.announce`	Yes
Behavioral medicine discussion	`alt.med.behavioral`	No
Cognitive science	`sci.cognitive`	No
Consciousness	`sci.psychology.consciousness`	Yes
Jung, Carl	`alt.psychology.jung`	No
Medicine, general	`sci.med`	No
Mental health as viewed in society	`alt.society.mental-health`	No
Neurolinguistic Programming (NLP)	`alt.psychology.nlp`	No
Nursing topics	`sci.med.nursing`	No
Personality	`sci.psychology.personality`	No
Personality models and assessment measures (such as Myers–Briggs)	`alt.psychology.personality`	No
Psyche, an electronic journal	`sci.psychology.journals.psyche`	Yes
Psychobiology and psychiatry	`sci.med.psychobiology`	No
Psychological research	`sci.psychology.research`	Yes
Psychological theory	`sci.psychology.theory`	No
Psychology, general	`sci.psychology.misc`	No
Psychotherapy	`sci.psychology.psychotherapy`	No
Psychotherapy, moderated	`sci.psychology.psychotherapy.moderated`	Yes
Psycoloquy, an electronic journal	`sci.psychology.journals.psycoloquy`	Yes
Research discussion	`sci.research`	No
Transpersonal psychology	`alt.psychology.transpersonal`	No

CAN I FIND A COLLEAGUE'S REAL-WORLD OR E-MAIL ADDRESS THROUGH MY COMPUTER?

There are several Web sites that will allow you to quickly and easily locate lost colleagues, friends, and even family members. There are databases of national White Page directories and e-mail directories. I list four of them. None of these directories is 100% accurate or complete, and there is no guarantee that you will actually locate the person you're searching for in this manner. White Page listings are restricted to public listings; these online services will not find private listings. Many of the services listed below also note people who use a certain type of Internet telephone software (also known as "NetPhones," see Chapter 10).

Most of the following services require that you know, accurately, the person's first and last names. So if you're not sure how to spell someone's name, you should try a several spellings and consider using a "wildcard" operator.

Title (or descriptor):	Yahoo! People Search
Owner:	Yahoo!, Inc.
URL (Web address):	`http://people.yahoo.com/`
Rating:	★★★
Access restrictions:	Registration is optional; free

After Yahoo! gobbled up the accurate online white pages directory Four11 in 1998, the quality of their people-finding database dropped drastically. Nowadays, however, Yahoo! has managed to regain the currency of its white pages address directory. People Search consistently found the current addresses of people I typed into it, although the information wasn't always correct. On the e-mail search component, however, Yahoo! couldn't find even my e-mail address, which hasn't changed for years. Because Yahoo! is a commercial online service, it also places additional lookup services on the same page as its free search service. This sponsorship placement (which is noted in small typeface) could be confusing to users who are confronted with a multitude of fields they can type into. Stick to the Yahoo! People Search table for the free and fairly accurate white page results.

Title (or descriptor):	Infospace
Owner:	Infospace
URL (Web address):	`http://www.infospace.com/`
Rating:	★★

Greatly diversifying its online offerings, Infospace's telephone, e-mail, and NetPhone directories are only a small part of its online community. Unfortunately, the quality of its directories seem to suffer as a result. Like Yahoo!'s People Search, it supports searching for people's (again, in separate databases, which makes searches unnecessary repetitive and time consuming) telephone numbers, e-mail addresses, and Net-Phones (found, cryptically, under the Net Community listing). The database also supports reverse lookups, a feature which allows you to find a person at a particular phone number. It offers business Yellow Pages as well, to help find a business in your local area. Infospace often returned no results on e-mail searches, or the wrong contact information altogether. It also failed to list people whose names approximate your name query, in case you spelled it wrong. For searching for people in the real world (e.g., physical addresses), Infospace's White Pages would appear to net you better results (although it still failed to find some people I threw at it). But for online connections, you would be better off using another directory service.

Title (or descriptor):	Switchboard
Owner:	Switchboard
URL (Web address):	`http://www.switchboard.com/`
Rating:	★★★

Switchboard is a directory for searching for real-world phone numbers and addresses of both individuals and businesses. I found its listings to be the most accurate and up-to-date database available online today, finding address changes made within the past year. Its database of e-mail addresses, however, was much less accurate and should not be used.

Title (or descriptor):	WhoWhere?
Owner:	Lycos?
URL (Web address):	`http://whowhere.lycos.com/`
Rating:	★★

Like all the other directory services online today, WhoWhere has branched out into creating an online community. If you thought its acquition by Lycos would help increase the resources devoted to keeping its directories accurate and up-to-date, you would be wrong. The quality of their directory is no better than any other directory reviewed, with out-of-date listings and no entries for over 60% of the people I typed in. The search capabilities are flexible, however, allowing you to search on a whole name or parts of a name. Unlike other directories, more results were often returned (even if many of them were inaccurate).

HOW DO I FIND COLLEAGUES AROUND THE WORLD WHO ARE DOING SIMILAR TYPES OF RESEARCH?

Academicians who do research in a particular subcategory of psychology have typically become aware of colleagues with similar research interests through a perusal of the psychological research literature. This works relatively well because professionals with research interests in a specific subject matter generally publish in regular peer-reviewed journals. But, this method also has its drawbacks. New researchers are more difficult to locate, since they may have no publications under their belt. Becoming published in a peer-reviewed, academic journal is an arduous and usually lengthy process. This is off-putting to some researchers who simply choose not to publish significant findings, or do so in nontraditional media (such as online). A fair amount of relevant and useful research also will be rejected from such journals, because of the peer-review process or stringent publishing standards. Many clinicians simply forgo the process of publishing their case studies and research findings altogether, because of the inherent difficulty in doing so and the time required to write up their results. Nonetheless, all of these professionals may still want to share and discuss their findings with other interested professionals around the world.

There are a number online methods that can help researchers and others interested in a specific research question find one another more quickly and easily. One method, detailed in the Step-by-Step box, is to submit an announcement about your research interests or findings to a professional mailing list or newsgroup. Another method is to examine journals' Web sites (whether they are electronic journals or otherwise) and browse through the research articles (see Chapter 9). Other methods might include browsing through some Web sites that offer databases of research in progress or researchers' field of study (see later in this section). All of these methods suffer from the same problem: the majority of professionals are not yet connected to the online world. The sample, therefore, is likely to be quite small compared to what a researcher may discover in the real world. This problem will naturally decrease in time.

Browsing through Journals' Web Sites

A second potentially useful method of finding colleagues is to examine the journals' Web sites (see Chapter 9) and read through research articles online. This can be more painstaking, because the only sure-fire method of ensuring your search is accurate and complete is to visit each journal and Web site. Why? Because search engines are having an increasingly harder time keeping up with the growth and volume of the World Wide Web. Search engines also may not index new articles and research for months after they've been online.

Searching through Online Databases and Search Engines

A less-painful means of locating research and current studies being conducted (and the people behind them) is through a clinical trials listing service, such as CenterWatch (listed below). Another means is looking through a database of clinicians or using an Internet search engine.

Using an Internet search engine to find colleagues is fairly simple. It does, however, require that the researcher or clinician you are searching for has what's known as an "online footprint." This means that the individual has some information published about him or her online. This is not always the case, and so Internet search engines, like all such methods, are not the most reliable.

To use a search engine to find a colleague, all you need to do is to form a query that matches your interests. For example, if you were a cognitive-behavioral researcher interested in the efficacy of cognitive-behavioral therapy, you might type in a Google query similar to:

```
"cognitive behavioral" researcher psychotherapy
```

Keywords such as "investigator," "clinical," "psychologist," "therapist," or "grant" might also be helpful to track down individuals associated with your field of interest.

STEP-BY-STEP: PUBLISHING THE ANNOUNCEMENT

1. Choose an appropriate mailing list or newsgroup. I recommend one of the following:

A. Mailing lists:

- ■ PsyUSA (see page 152)
- ■ Clinical psychologists (see pages 151–152)

B. Newsgroups:

- ■ `sci.psychology.research` (moderated)
- ■ `sci.med.psychobiology`

2. Write a short paragraph that briefly describes your active research interests, the findings of a study, or a case study you'd like to share with other professionals. Be sure to include a good subject line for your article. For example:

Subject: Cognitive Elaboration Rating System compiled

My name is John Grohol and I'm a psychologist interested in the cognitive elaboration model of psychotherapy interactions. I recently helped compile a rating system with some colleagues of mine to measure and record therapist–client interactions in a given therapy session. I would be happy to discuss and share this new rating system with anyone who might be interested in psychotherapy outcome research. Please e-mail me at `grohol@psychcentral.com` for additional information or questions.

Title (or descriptor):	CenterWatch
Owner:	CenterWatch, Inc.
URL (Web address):	`http://www.centerwatch.com/`
Rating:	★★★★

Important points to consider:

■ Do not submit an entire study to a mailing list or newsgroup. (One exception is the `sci.psychology.research` newsgroup, which does accept completed studies for publication online.) You should keep the announcement short and to the point, giving readers all the relevant information they need to know about your interests in one or two paragraphs.

■ Do not submit your announcement to mailing lists or newsgroups where such submissions may be frowned upon. When in doubt, contact the mailing list's owner or administrator before making the submission and ask for permission.

■ Space your announcement submissions so that you don't barrage all the mailing lists and newsgroups at once. Such a barrage is frowned on in the online world. Post to no more than two mailing lists at a time, and not more than a half-dozen newsgroups. Wait a week and then post to another two mailing lists, if need be. While newsgroups have a much wider readership than most mailing lists, their readers tend to be laypeople rather than fellow professionals.

■ Do not keep submit your announcements more than once every 6 months or so. Mailing list and newsgroup readers do not change that drastically from month to month.

■ If you get no response from this method, you might try looking for more specific and appropriate mailing lists or discussion forums in which to publish your announcement. It may also be that there is no one else subscribed to that mailing list or newsgroup who is interested in your research subject matter.

■ If all else fails, try another method outlined in this section.

This the central clinical trials listing service online, offering researchers and clinicians descriptions of current research. Listings are arranged by general medical specialty (psychiatry/psychology being of interest to us), and within each specialty by disorder under study. Choosing a disorder gives you the name of the center or agency conducting the study, arranged by states, as well as a brief one-line description of the study. By clicking on the center's name, you may get additional information and details on the study as well as a contact person for the research. While this database is targeted toward participants, researchers may use it as well to discover current research being conducted. The Web site is well designed and easy to understand.

Title (or descriptor):   Who's Who in Mental Health on the Web
Owner: Linda M. Chapman, MSW, LCSW
URL (Web address):   `http://wwmhw.com/`
Rating: ★★★

Who's Who in Mental Health on the Web is a professional database currently listing over 2,200 mental health professionals' networking and practice interests. Any mental health professional can register with the database at no charge, and list their contact information and research, practice and networking interests within their entry. A search engine makes the database easy to use. Type in keywords—such as "cognitive research"—into the search box first. Then choose the option, "Find all of these words" to get the best results from the search engine.

CHAPTER 7

Researching Online: References and Databases

Entire books have been written about how to effectively conduct research and literature searches online. The truth of the matter is, though, that useful research discovery, references, abstracts, and information are rarely fully realized through simply getting online and browsing the World Wide Web. Serious researchers will still conduct their literature searches, for the most part, in a library, because libraries still easily outperform the online world in the depth and breadth of information available. And until every book and journal is converted into an electronic format, libraries will remain the gold standard and preferred option for conducting literature searches and doing background research.

However, you can do background research through online resources. But the quality and quantity of work you will find online will vary greatly, depending on the specific topic under study. For instance, in studying depression and looking for related statistics of this disorder for your research, you will probably find the needed information at the National Institute of Mental Health (`http://www.nimh.nih.gov/`). What you will not find, however, are references or abstracts to the majority of the social science literature done on this topic in the past decade. You can find a fair amount of medically related literature on it, through a MEDLINE search or a summary article written by a psychiatrist (see, for example, Internet Mental Health at `http://www.mentalhealth.com/`). But such information is very limited in its scope and excludes the bulk of relevant literature, such as that found in psychology, sociology, social psychology, cognitive science, and epidemiology. Topics that are even less well known (for instance, a paper about John Dewey) will probably garner even less useful information. The library is still the best place to begin and end such a search. It will probably remain so for at least the near future.

However, there can be useful aspects to online research searches. It may help you refine and better define your research ideas or hypotheses. It may also help you to look up information on topics related to your original idea that you may not have thought of to begin with. Such online research also has the potential to put you in touch with other researchers or professionals interested in ideas and topic areas similar to your own. Collaboration or at least the ability to bounce ideas off of these like-minded professionals can be accomplished through such communication.

Many professionals' current use of computer technology is limited to literature searches or similar uses to find specific information in a reference database. PsycINFO is the most popular and probably well-known example of a research database, because today's professionals used it extensively in their graduate studies. MEDLINE is another such database, as is the ERIC catalog of academic articles and papers. While these were, at one time, only available in paper format, they have long since become electronic because of the computer's ability to search through thousands of abstracts quickly for key terms or search queries. Much like Web-based search engines, all of these databases rely on a similar piece of software to index the catalog to allow for easy and fast searches on it.

It would make sense, then, that if these databases are already computerized, they should be available for searching online. All of them are, and most of them are available at the present time without cost. Examples of free databases include ERIC and MEDLINE at the present time; PsycINFO is available at costs that vary from vendor to vendor. These fees may change as the American Psychological Association looks to become more competitive with similar types of databases available without charge online. It is just as possible that other vendors will begin charging for those databases that are currently available at no charge. Ultimately, the market (i.e., you) will decide what it is and is not willing to pay for online.

Diagnosis and medication are categories of reference material commonly used by both clinicians and researchers. Both of these categories, in many different forms and formats, are available online from a wide variety of sites. Some material will include much the same information found in real-world reference manuals, either quoted from that material or written from scratch, because of copyright restrictions.

HOW DO I LOCATE THE RESEARCH AND CLINICAL ABSTRACT DATABASES—SUCH AS ERIC, MEDLINE, AND PsycINFO?

Below are some of the places where you can go online to find these databases. If you're looking for a journal's Web site, please refer to Chapter 9.

ERIC

Title (or descriptor):	ERIC Clearinghouse on Assessment and Evaluation
Owner:	U.S. Department of Education
URL (Web address):	http://www.ericae.net/
URL (Web address):	http://www.eric.ed.gov/
Rating:	★★★

The Educational Resources Information Center (ERIC), as noted on their Web site, is

> a national information system designed to provide users with ready access to an extensive body of education-related literature. ERIC, established in 1966, is supported by the U.S. Department of Education, Office of Educational Research and Improvement, and the National Library of Education. . . . The database contains more than 850,000 abstracts of documents and journal articles on education research and practice.

The Web site provides direct online and free access to the ERIC database since 1991 (although other online ERIC databases back to 1989 are also available and accessible through this Web site). You can also fill out a document-ordering form to obtain documents you find within the database. The Web site allows readers to locate citations and reviews of educational and psychological tests and measures that The Buros Institute of Mental Measurements and ProEd (a book publisher) have included in their directories. The Web site is well designed, although the graphics look a little cheesy. This site is a good example of the power of putting database resources online, especially for researchers.

MEDLINE

MEDLINE is the medical abstract research database roughly equivalent to PsycLIT for psychology. Always available to physicians and medical students at no charge, it is now available to anyone online to search through for free. It can be accessed through a variety of Web sites. Some of these sites also offer document retrieval delivered to your home or office for a fee. MEDLINE contains over 9 million references from over 3,900 journals, and includes abstracts from the vast majority of the social sciences and psychology literature. It can be used as a free alternative to the PsycINFO products from the American Psychological Association.

Title (or descriptor):	Community of Science MEDLINE
Owner:	Community of Science, Inc.
URL (Web address):	`http://medline.cos.com/`
Rating:	★★
Access restrictions:	Registration required; fees variable

The Community of Science dropped its free MEDLINE searches and now makes its database available only to paid subscribers. Subscriptions start at $175/year for individuals. Three search forms offer the user a wide variety of options to choose from in forming everything from a quick and simple query, to a complex and detailed query.

Title (or descriptor):	Infotrieve MEDLINE Service Provider
Owner:	Infotrieve, Inc.

URL (Web address): `http://www4.infotrieve.com/`
Rating: ★★

Another free MEDLINE search service, which gives you the ability to form natural language or Boolean queries, which ever you prefer. Offers TOXLINE and AIDSLINE access in addition to advanced search functions. The full text of articles is available for between $12.00 and $24.00, plus copyright fees (typically $2–$30 per article).

Title (or descriptor): Medscape MEDLINE Search
Owner: Medscape
URL (Web address): `http://www.medscape.com/`
Rating: ★★★
Access restrictions: Free registration required

Utilizing the full MEDLINE database (from 1966 to the present) along with an easy registration process and free searches helps make this one of the stonger MEDLINE search sites. The full text of articles is available by mail for $8.00 plus copyright fees. Results are displayed in order of relevance, and, unlike on government sites, advertisements are found on every page.

Title (or descriptor): NLM Gateway
Owner: National Library of Medicine
URL (Web address): `http://gateway.nlm.nih.gov/`
Rating: ★★★

A new service from the National Library of Medicine, the NLM Gateway allows a user to search multiple databases simultaneously, including MEDLINE (medical and social science journal citations, 1966 to present), OLDMEDLINE (medical and social science journal citations, 1958–1965), LOCATORplus (catalog records for book, serials, audiovisual materials), AIDS meetings (meeting abstracts on AIDS/HIV), Health Services Research meetings, HSRProj (health services research projects in progress), MEDLINEplus (general information on health topics), and DIRLINE (directory of health organizations). By typing in just a few keywords, NLM Gateway returns a list of items found, sorted into major categories: journal citations, books/serials/AVs, general consumer health, meeting abstracts, and other collections. It is well organized and easy to use, offering a one-stop search interface for the researcher, professional, and consumer to a number of major U.S. federal government databases.

Title (or descriptor):	PaperChase
Owner:	PaperChase
URL (Web address):	`http://www.paperchase.com/`
Rating:	★★
Access restrictions:	Registration required; free trial or $150.00/year

It is questionable whether the cost of viewing abstracts through PaperChase is offset by its interactive search designed for beginners. The search feature on PaperChase is designed to help a user narrow their chosen topics in order to provide more relevant results. This may be helpful to new users, but will likely impede and frustrate experienced users. The Web site becomes confused if your try and take a shortcut by using the built-in history function of your Web browser, so you are forced to use the site's own navigation tools (another drawback to its design). The search recognizes only Boolean queries. Before using the free trial, users are requested to fill out a registration form. There is apparently no way to order the full text of articles.

Title (or descriptor):	PubMed
Owner:	National Library of Medicine
URL (Web address):	`http://www.ncbi.nlm.nih.gov/PubMed/`
Rating:	★★★★

PubMed acts as the gold standard of MEDLINE databases. It is free, the most updated, and easiest site to use to access the current MEDLINE database. Maintained by the same folks who maintain the actual MEDLINE database, the PubMed Web site is easy to use for beginners, but also offers a mix of advanced features for more experienced researchers. Unlike some of the commercial services, however, you cannot simply order a copy of an article off its Web site (it's more complicated than that on PubMed). For experienced researchers affiliated with a university, or others that live nearby a university library, the lack of this ordering ability is not a serious detriment, as the journals are usually readily available for lookup.

PsycINFO

Title (or descriptor):	American Psychological Association
Owner:	American Psychological Association
URL (Web address):	`http://www.apa.org/psycinfo/`
Rating:	★★★

After years of outsourcing direct access to its PsycINFO database, the American Psychological Association has finally provided individuals a way to access it directly. Anybody can access it for $11.95 for 24 hours, or members of the APA who already subscribe to any APA journal can gain full access to the database for an entire year for $139.00. These rates are less expensive than access to PsycINFO from a third-party provider (listed below), because there is no per-record viewing or downloading charge. If you do not have access to PsycINFO via a university affiliation, this is the most inexpensive and fastest way to obtain such access.

For most academicians and students, such services, while convenient, are probably not very cost-effective. The databases are often found at educational institutions and are available to faculty and students free of charge. Many universities also make them available through their own local computer network on campus, but only if you are a current student or faculty member. Using the university's existing PsycINFO database is usually cheaper and may be accessible via your university's local computer network, which you can confirm by contacting the reference librarian in the university library. The librarian can also provide you with instructions on how to access the database directly. Alternatively, some university libraries and departments offer search services for faculty and students, often for a fee.

If you don't have convenient, free access to these databases through an academic institution, you can still find them online for a fee. American Psychological Association (APA) members can subscribe to PsycINFO access as a part of their membership benefits. Other options for individual access to the service are available at:

`http://www.apa.org/psycinfo/products/individuals.html`

For example, the APA offers direct access to the database for 24 hours for a flat fee of $11.95 with unlimited searches and download of abstracts. This is probably the most economical and simple way to access the database on a moment's notice. Other service plans are available on their Web site.

I'M DOING RESEARCH ON A SPECIFIC TOPIC— HOW DO I FIND INFORMATION ONLINE ABOUT IT?

There are two methods you can use to find research online. One method is to search specialized indices for research papers, such as those listed later in this section. But perhaps the easier and more common method is by beginning with a powerful search engine such as Google (`http://www.google.com/`) or a meta-search engine such as Vivismo (`http://www.vivisimo.com/`), as described in the Step-by-Step box.

Another, less-useful method to finding research online is to visit one of the many research archives. These reside at a number of different Web sites, and are specific to specialized research topics. In most cases, this method won't be that helpful unless you just happen to need to find research on one of these topic areas. Unfortunately, at the present time, there is no central online clearinghouse or index for such papers. You should also keep in mind the vast number of journals that host Web sites; research articles may often be found there too.

Title (or descriptor):	HeartMath Research Papers
Owner:	Institute of HeartMath
URL (Web address):	`http://www.heartmath.org/`
Rating:	★★

The Institute of HeartMath is a nonprofit institution, whose research division's mission is to explore the central role of the heart's electrical system in health and well-being. A number of research papers are available through this site on these topics.

STEP-BY-STEP: FINDING RELEVANT RESEARCH ONLINE

1. Select a search engine or a meta-search engine (for example, AltaVista or Inference Find).

2. Keep your initial query as general as possible.

3. Submit multiple queries, adding additional keywords, operators, or search terms in different combinations and phrases as needed to narrow your search. Here are some examples.

Task: Find information on the cognitive elaboration likelihood model

Step 1. Choose a search engine, such as Google.

Step 2. Form an initial, general query. I'll start with the phrase `"cognitive elaboration"` (with the quotes).

Step 3. If too many irrelevant results are obtained, resubmit the query, adding another word to the phrase. In my example, I'll add the word "likelihood" and resubmit the query as the phrase, `"cognitive elaboration likelihood"`.

Task: Find information on Prozac (fluoxetine) efficacy versus other treatment

Step 1. Choose a search engine.

Step 2. Form an initial, general query. I'll start with the query: `prozac OR fluoxetine`

Step 3. This brings up far too many results. So I'll narrow my search by adding some additional operators and a word: `(prozac OR fluoxetine) efficacy`

Task: Use Google's "Advanced Search" features to limit the results of the above example

Step 1. Using Google, choose the "Advanced Search" option.

Step 2. Form the initial query in the "Find results with all the words" field. In that box, I'll enter our last query: `(prozac OR fluoxetine) efficacy`. You can choose additional options on this page, such as limiting the results to return only pages in English (or another language of your choosing) and only pages updated in the past 3 or 6 months. This helps to ensure that your results are not only relevant, but timely as well.

Step 3. If you are still sifting through too many irrelevant results, there are additional fields in the "Find results" table that you can add words to, including specific phrases and additional words that must also appear on the page. For instance, I might add the word `research` to appear in our results. You can also easily add words from the "Advanced Search" function that you don't want appearing in your results, in case you are finding a common but irrelevant term appearing over and over again. If I kept finding results mentioning a type of treatment program, I might put the word `program` in the field of words I don't want appearing in my results.

Title (or descriptor):	ingenta
Owner:	ingenta
URL (Web address):	`http://www.ingenta.com/`
Rating:	★★

Ingenta, which merged with UnCover in 2000, attempts to provide a single point of access for researchers and professionals in every scientific field. With such a broad mission, it is not surprising that it has difficulty in fulfilling its mission for each specific field. A search through Uncover plus returns far fewer results (and often, less relevant results) than a search through MEDLINE.

Title (or descriptor):	Journal of Neurotherapy
Owner:	Society for Neuronal Regulation
URL (Web address):	`http://www.snr-jnt.org/`
Rating:	★★★

An interesting site with dozens of articles online taken directly from the *Journal of Neurotherapy*. Most of the peer-reviewed articles cover topics such as EEG biofeedback and neurofeedback, the focus of the journal and society. One of the oldest such repositories online, and still updated regularly.

Medscape

Title (or descriptor):	Medscape Psychiatry & Mental Health
Owner:	WebMD, Inc.
URL (Web address):	`http://www.medscape.com/psychiatryhome/`
Rating:	★★★★

A growing repository of respectable, peer-reviewed articles in psychiatry and mental health are available at no charge from Medscape. Topics range from detailed discussions regarding the latest treatment options for specific disorders, to trends in psychopharmacological treatment and prevention. Psychiatry news, conference summaries, and practice guidelines round out this excellent resource for therapists. Overseen by a scientific advisory board led by Charles L. Bowden, M.D. and 11 other physicians, the site's central drawback is its medical focus and orientation.

Title (or descriptor):	Mental Help Net Professional Resources
Owner:	CenterSite, LLC
URL (Web address):	`http://mentalhelp.net/`
Rating:	★★

Divided by broad topic areas, each page in the professional resources section of this Web site includes a category for journals and research papers online. While probably not a comprehensive index, it may be a good place to browse through some research archives on a variety of professional topic areas, such as alcoholism and substance abuse, cognitive and behavioral therapy, health and sports psychology, industrial and organizational psychology, and others.

Title (or descriptor):	Prevention and Treatment
Owner:	American Psychological Association
URL (Web address):	`http://journals.apa.org/prevention/`
Rating:	★★

An electronic-only journal that got off to a rocky start, it has irregular articles on varying psychological topics. These topics range from efficacy and outcome research in psychotherapy, to an analysis of drug treatment outcomes. At this point, the emphasis seems to be on treatment, not prevention. A sampling of some of the most recent articles in the journal, three were reprints from other sources, and a portion of the fourth appeared in another publication. But commentaries accompanying each article are original to the journal.

Title (or descriptor):	PubMed Central
Owner:	National Institutes of Health
URL (Web address):	`http://www.pubmedcentral.nih.gov/`
Rating:	Unrated

PubMed Central is a new service of the U.S. National Institutes of Health (NIH). PubMed Central is "a Web-based repository for barrier-free access to primary reports in the life sciences. [. . .] PubMed Central will archive, organize and distribute peer-reviewed reports from journals, as well as reports that have been screened but not formally peer-reviewed," according to the NIH. It will be interesting to see if this concept turns into an evolution in scientific publishing.

GRANT SEARCHES ONLINE

Grant searching can now largely be conducted online. While a search at your local university library will still likely yield researchers more results, online grant searchers can be a helpful place to start. Many Web sites, especially federal government resources, allow you to download the grant applications online. Most such applications, to retain their original formatting, are available in *PDF* format. A PDF viewer, which allow you to view and print out PDF documents, is available for free from Adobe's Web site (`http://www.adobe.com/`).

Title:	APA Research Awards
Owner:	American Psychiatric Association
URL:	`http://www.psych.org/res_res/awards.cfm`
Rating:	★★

Provides application guidelines for a handful of psychiatric and psychobiological research awards. Most of the grants listed are funded by pharmaceutical companies.

Title:	DHHS GrantsNet
Owner:	U.S. Department of Health and Human Services (DHHS)
URL:	`http://www.hhs.gov/grantsnet/`
Rating:	★★

A basic U.S. government Web site which offers a limited amount of information and links to funding opportunities online. It is not clear how often the site is updated, and the links to actual DHHS funding information were difficult to find and navigate. This was due in part to the site's reliance on the older gopher file and retrieval system (which has largely been superseced by the World Wide Web).

Title:	The Foundation Center Online
Owner:	The Foundation Center
URL:	`http://fdncenter.org/`
Rating:	★★★★

Whether you're an experienced or beginner grant-seeker, the Foundation Center Online is an invaluable resource. The Foundation Center is **the** resource for grant writing, publishing *FC Search: The Foundation Center's Database on CD-ROM*. This database, while not available for searching from their Web site, is available for purchase or access at no charge within over 200 libraries throughout the United States. The database acts as a comprehensive starting point for anyone interested in grant funding for their research, program, or nonprofit organization. The Foundation Center's Web site offers users practically every piece of information related to grant writing except this database. Extensive, well-written tutorials help first-time grant authors understand the process and walks them through it, step by step. Additional resources include additional information about the Foundation, funding trends and analysis (including the U.S.'s top corporate funders), and a complete searchable archive and current issue of *Philanthropy News Digest*.

Title:	Grants Central
Owner:	Polaris Services
URL:	`http://polarisgrantscentral.net/`
Rating:	★★

Generally an annotated list of real-world references and resources which may be of value to grant writers. Polaris is a company which helps train individuals through publications and workshops on the subject of grants acquisition.

Title:	GrantsNet
Owner:	American Association for the Advancement of Science
URL:	http://www.grantsnet.org/
Rating:	★★★

This Web site, updated regularly, offers funding opportunities for training in the biological and medical sciences. While not offering a whole lot of funding opportunities for the behavioral health professions, some researchers may find the grants listed useful to their research. The site sports a fullly searchable database of over 200 programs. Regularly updated funding news is a helpful aid to keep on top of emerging funding opportunities. Nearly 700 organizations' names and contact information are listed in their funding directory. This site is attractively designed and simple to navigate, although a one-time, free registration is required to access their datebase.

Title:	NIH Grants Information
Owner:	National Institutes of Health (NIH)
URL:	http://grants.nih.gov/grants/
Rating:	★★★

The National Institutes of Health (NIH) offers one of the most comprehensive and useful online databases for federal funding opportunities. The NIH is also one of the few sites which actually allows you to search (via a powerful and useful search engine) for grants based upon keywords, research interests, or topics. The Guide for Grants and Contracts, as NIH calls its grants database, is also browseable by date. Users may also subscribe to a free mailing list which notifies recipients of changes made to the grants database every week. The two biggest drawbacks to the database is that out-dated grant announcements are not removed from it and that the text of the announcements is lengthy and poorly formatted (it is, therefore, best printed out). The NIH should sort out archival announcements from current announcements to aid grant seekers. As with nearly any government program, a great deal of the documentation associated with NIH grants is lengthy and complex. This includes not only NIH's introductory information to grant writing and submissions, but also its frequently asked questions article. The search help was not customized to reflect the content and queries users of the NIH site are likely to form. This made it difficult to determine how best to form a useful query. For those with experience in obtaining NIH grants, the site will be a valuable resource offering tools and aid in their funding quest. For those with lesser grant experience, the site may be confusing and difficult to navigate.

Title:	NIMH Grants
Owner:	National Institute of Mental Health (NIMH)
URL:	`http://www.nimh.nih.gov/grants/index.cfm`
Rating:	★★★

Information related to research, research training and career development, and special program grants and funding opportunitites are available from the NIMH'a site. Updated regularly, the resources on the site are logically organized and are simple to navigate. A lengthy introductory article about NIMH grants is especially useful to first-time grant authors.

Title:	Office of Research, Health Sciences
Owner:	University of Pittsburgh
URL:	`http://www.oorhs.pitt.edu/`
Rating:	★★

The Office of Research, Health Sciences (OORHS) "nurtures research activities in the health sciences by providing support for the specialized needs of biomedical researchers" for the University of Pittsburgh. This site provides an up-to-date listing of funding opportunities related to the university.

Professional Associations, Issues, and Ethics Online

Some of the best-designed and most informative Web sites online today are those created by specific professional associations. You will discover not only information related to professional issues and ethics on such sites, but membership information, contacts for the organization, calendars of workshops and events, lists of online resources, and a good deal more. Naturally, some association Web sites are more helpful than others. In general, the larger the organization the more complete the Web site.

WHAT ARE SOME IMPORTANT ETHICAL CONCERNS FOR PROFESSIONALS ONLINE?

Ethics are an important aspect of any profession. They are especially vital to the helping professions where individuals are often in emotional distress and therefore are more vulnerable. The application of ethical and professional standards to the online world is still in its formative stages. Many professional organizations are not yet certain how to translate real-world ethics to the electronic, "virtual" world. The larger professional organizations, such as the American Psychological Association and American Psychiatric Association, are taking conservative, wait-and-see stances. In the meantime, there are some unique issues I'll address in this chapter, which are not likely to be specifically addressed in any profession's ethical code or guidelines. But these issues are *vitally important* for you to understand and consider as you engage in any type of online interaction. They concern confidentiality, informed consent, and conducting therapy over the Internet.

Confidentiality Online

A special concern in the online world is confidentiality of a client's personal background and history. Just as in the real world, professionals must use care when presenting a case on a mailing list (or any other online discussion forum). Information published on the mailing list will reach hundreds, potentially thousands, of others across the world, and there is no guarantee that all of them will be professionals or bound by any ethical code of conduct. Identifying information must be left out or changed; this includes geographical locations and names of significant others in relation to the client. Professionals should never assume that because they subscribe to a professional mailing list, it is safe to discuss cases as they would in an office with the door closed. *Mailing lists are public forums*—only slightly less public than other forums online (such as newsgroups or Web-based discussion areas). In other words, exercise the same care as you would if you were presenting the case to the entire staff of your clinic or hospital. This will ensure the patient's confidentiality is not compromised as well as maintain your professional ethics and image.

Informed Consent

There are other professional issues in dealing with ordinary people in the online world. Some researchers have engaged in ethically questionable behavior online by conducting naturalistic studies through observation of a support mailing list or newsgroup. These researchers did not gain the mailing list users' consent, nor did the users have any reason to expect that their interactions on the mailing list would come under scrutiny or be used as an object of study. I find the downside of such research to far outweigh any benefits. A few months back, someone sent me e-mail about this situation. A researcher was discussing the results of such a study to a large audience. Unknown to the researcher, one of the mailing list's participants was sitting in the audience. She was aghast to discover that her behaviors on the list had been studied and were now being presented to a large group of complete strangers!

Should such naturalistic research take place online? Yes, if it is conducted in the same manner that real-world naturalistic studies are—with full consensual participation by those being observed. This question was answered long ago in the real world. Just because the modality of communication has changed doesn't mean that researchers and professionals are no longer bound by the same ethical principles.

Therapy over the Internet

Another hot ethical issue is the question of conducting psychotherapy online. This question has remained largely unresolved in any codified fashion to this point. For a longer discussion of the ethical and professional issues in conducting online therapy, as well as resources offering more information, see Chapter 11. For now, suffice to say that you should think long and hard before hanging out your virtual shingle.

ARE THE ETHICAL PRINCIPLES FOR VARIOUS MENTAL HEALTH PROFESSIONS AVAILABLE ONLINE?

Yes, most such ethical principles and guidelines are available online. For ethical guidelines, the logical place to look is the appropriate professional association that writes or oversees such guidelines. For psychologists, it's the

American Psychological Association; for psychiatrists, it's the American Psychiatric Association. Other professions may also find their ethical codes online at their respective national association's Web site. State licensing in the United States doesn't require a professional to be a member of a professional guild, nor do states have their own individual ethical principles (although they often adopt the professional association's guidelines by law). So such principles may apply to practicing professionals in their respective fields in the United States, but not necessarily to international psychologists or psychiatrists.

Title (or descriptor):   American Counseling Association

Owner: American Counseling Association

URL (Web address):

    `http://www.counseling.org/site/`
    `PageServer?pagename=resources_ethics`

Rating: ★★★

The code of ethics for counselors may be found here, available as one large file (which will take most computers a few minutes to load). Use your Web browser's "Find" function (often found under the "Edit" menu) to locate specific areas of interest, or use the index at the top of the document to jump down to major categories. The "Standards of Practice" for counselors are a part of this same document, as are references for the entire document. No frequently asked questions (FAQ) file on how to report ethics violations is available.

Title (or descriptor):   American Psychiatric Association–Membership Ethics

Owner: American Psychiatric Association

URL (Web address):

    `http://www.psych.org/apa_members/ethics.cfm`

Rating: ★★★

The "Principles of Medical Ethics" make up the bulk of the content of this section within the American Psychiatric Association's Web site. The APA has adopted and annotated the American Medical Association's medical ethics to make them more applicable and relevant to psychiatry. The original and the annotated versions are available here, as are the procedure used for filing a complaint against a psychiatrist member and an FAQ file about how ethical complaints are handled. The information appears current and is certainly relevant to professionals within the psychiatric field. This section suffers from the same problem as the rest of the APA Web site, as I'll discuss in more detail later in this chapter—it is too hierarchical in structure. Finding relevant items often requires exploring layers upon layers of menu lists.

Title (or descriptor):	American Psychological Association–Ethics Information
Owner:	American Psychological Association
URL (Web address):	http://www.apa.org/ethics/
Rating:	★★★

The information found here could certainly be more online-friendly, as they have placed the entire listing of ethical principles into one, very large file. The same is true of the APA Ethics Committee Rules and Procedures, whose file is even larger than the principles' file itself. (If that isn't a comment about bureaucracy, I don't know what is!). The authors have at least taken the time to properly convert the ethical principles into a Web-based format so you can jump around in the large document relatively easily. Unlike the American Psychiatric Association, there is no FAQ file so members who have a complaint filed against them or are seeking to file an ethics complaint won't really know what to expect unless they call the APA directly. Statements about telephone and online therapy as well as behavioral research with animals may also be found here, as are guidelines for ethical conduct in the care and use of animals.

Title (or descriptor):	National Association of Social Workers–Code of Ethics
Owner:	National Association of Social Workers (NASW)
URL (Web address):	http://www.socialworkers.org/pubs/code/
Rating:	★★

Available directly from the Association's home page, the social workers' code of ethics is neatly organized. It is divided into a number of logical categories (preamble, purpose, ethical principles, and ethical standards). No FAQ file is available for consumers or professionals on how to resolve ethical dilemmas or complaints.

WHERE ARE THE PROFESSIONAL ASSOCIATIONS ONLINE?

There are a few places you can consult for indexes of professional organizations. One place might be to use Yahoo!'s (`http://www.yahoo.com/`) internal search engine to find such an organization quickly and easily (by just typing the association's name into the search query box). Another resource is Mental Health Net's (`http://mentalhelp.net/`) listing of professional associations and organizations under their "Professional Resources" category. Yet a third online listing of such resources is Myron Pulier's index (`http://www.umdnj.edu/psyevnts/psyjumps.html`). I've listed some of the larger organizations below in alphabetical order, for your convenience.

Title (or descriptor):	Albert Ellis Institute
Owner:	Albert Ellis Institute
URL (Web address):	`http://www.rebt.org/`
Rating:	★★★

This page provides a lot of useful information on rational emotive behavior therapy (REBT), a specific psychotherapy and theory developed by Albert Ellis. This Web site includes a directory of REBT-trained therapists throughout the world, an FAQ file, a schedule of upcoming seminars, and a host of other resources. It is interesting to discover that Albert Ellis answers one question a month posed to him by the public through this Web site. Who would have ever guessed that one of the pioneers in the field of psychotherapy could be found on the Web.

AMERICAN ACADEMY OF CHILD & ADOLESCENT PSYCHIATRY

AACAP

Title (or descriptor):	American Academy of Child and Adolescent Psychiatry
Owner:	American Academy of Child and Adolescent Psychiatry
URL (Web address):	`http://www.aacap.org/`
Rating:	★★★★

As noted on their Web site,

> The Academy represents over 6,500 child and adolescent psychiatrists—physicians with at least five years of additional training beyond medical school in

general and child and adolescent psychiatry. AACAP members actively research, diagnose and treat psychiatric disorders affecting children and adolescents and their families, and the Academy is dedicated to supporting this work through a variety of programs including government liaison, national public information and continuing medical education.

Their Web site reflects this dedication with sections for each of its offices. Offerings include one of the first online transplants of a helpful series of informational brochures called "Facts for Families." These brochures, available online and as regular printed publications in Spanish and French, provide concise and up-to-date material on issues ranging from children who suffer from depression and teen suicide, to stepfamily problems and child sexual abuse. It's usually a good recommendation to have parents read a relevant brochure if their child suffers from one of the topic areas covered. Press releases, legislative alerts, research and clinical information, and a calendar of events can all be found here. It has consistently been rated as one of the most popular and useful Web sites online today, which is probably due to its effective layout and easy navigation. Graphics are smaller once you get beyond the home page.

Title (or descriptor):	American Academy of Neurology (AAN)
Owner:	American Academy of Neurology
URL (Web address):	http://www.aan.com/
Rating:	★★★★

This Web site, providing information for both professionals and the public on neurology subjects, is large and very well designed. Once beyond the large graphics on the home page, pages are quick to load and attractively presented. The AAN is a professional organization representing neurologists worldwide. The Web site covers a multitude of information from Alzheimer's and Parkinson's diseases to stroke and migraine. Their comprehensive and well-written Fact Sheets cover topics such as Alzheimer's disease, anencephaly, Bell's palsy, boxing, brain tumors, carpal tunnel syndrome, chronic pain, epilepsy, tremor, headache, head injuries, lumbar puncture, multiple sclerosis, neuroaids, neuroimaging, Parkinson's disease, stroke, transient ischemic attack, Tourette's syndrome, and essential tremor; informational brochures on ALS and multiple sclerosis are also available. Information on neurology is also available, as is a "news" section, which highlights a different disorder every so often. This section also houses monthly news reports from the ANN journal, *Neurology*.

Title (or descriptor):	American Association for Emergency Psychiatry
Owner:	American Association for Emergency Psychiatry (AAEP)
URL (Web address):	`http://emergencypsychiatry.org/`
Rating:	★★

The American Association for Emergency Psychiatry (AAEP) is a multidisciplinary organization that provides a professional organizational voice in emergency mental health. The membership includes directors of psychiatric emergency services, psychiatrists, nurses, social workers, psychologists, physician assistants, educators, and other professionals involved in emergency psychiatry. The site is of basic design and functions for its intended purpose, but only provides the bare minimum in terms of information and resources. For instance, an index of articles for its journal is offered, but the articles themselves are not available online. Membership benefits, a membership form, and a meeting list round out the site.

Title (or descriptor):	American Association of Marriage and Family Therapy
Owner:	American Association of Marriage and Family Therapy
URL (Web address):	`http://www.aamft.org/`
Rating:	★★★

The American Association of Marriage and Family Therapy represents more than 23,000 marriage and family therapists throughout the world. Its site is a solid offering among professional associations, providing a good mix of membership and public information. The site is also home to TherapistLocator.net, a directory that lists a majority of its therapists allowing consumers to easily locate a marriage and family therapist within their local community. Consumer mental health information is readily available through a set of "Consumer Updates," online brochures written in down-to-earth language, on topics such as bereavement, children and divorce, domestic violence, infertility, as well as the more common mental health disorders. Conference announcements and organizational news are also available, as is a members-only area, which features jobs and peer networking resources.

Title (or descriptor):   American Association of Suicidology

Owner: American Association of Suicidology

URL (Web address):   `http://www.suicidology.org/`

Rating: ★★

The American Association of Suicidology (AAS) is a nonprofit organization dedicated to the understanding and prevention of suicide. Their site acts as a central online suicide resource not only for the association's members, but also professionals and laypeople. It is unfortunate that the site's design and layout are not exactly intuitive. Crisis centers are sorted only by state, which makes going through large states' listings a chore. (Hint: use your Web browser's within-page "Find" menu option.) The educational material on suicide is useful, and the members page succinctly describes the benefits of joining this organization.

Title (or descriptor):   American Board of Examiners in Clinical Social Work

Owner: American Board of Examiners (ABE)

URL (Web address):   `http://www.abecsw.org/`

Rating: ★★★

This Web site houses information about this organization, credentialing, ethics, and the board of directors. The American Board of Examiners (ABE) issues a credential—the Board Certified Diplomate in Clinical Social Work (BCD)—to advanced clinical social workers nationwide. Currently about 13,000 social workers hold this advanced credential. The site provides an online, searchable database of its members, making it easy to find professionals who hold the credential.

Title (or descriptor):   American Counseling Association

Owner: American Counseling Association

URL (Web address):   `http://www.counseling.org/`

Rating: ★★★★

This is an informative Web site offering a host of information about the American Counseling Association. In addition to offering general information about the association and membership, it hosts legislative and news updates, a conference and workshop calendar, as well as links to related resources and publications. *Counseling Today On-Line*, a monthly newsletter with informative articles and commentary, is also available. The code of ethics for counselors in addition to other professional information is offered. The Web site has reduced the use of overly large graphics over the years and now offers a relatively clean interface and faster Web site. The site is well designed and organized, but pages other than the home page lack information about when they were last updated.

Title (or descriptor):	American Medical Association
Owner:	American Medical Association
URL (Web address):	`http://www.ama-assn.org/`
Rating:	★★★★
Access restrictions:	Registration optional; free

The largest professional association of medical doctors in the world has a large and impressive Web site. It offers a wide range of medical information, links to their own journal (*Journal of the American Medical Association* [JAMA]), and links to a dozen other journals sponsored by the AMA, including the *Archives of General Psychiatry*. Full-text abstracts of each journal's current and past articles are available. Naturally information about the organization itself and its members is available. Advocacy, press releases, science, and education categories round out the site. Graphics are professional and usually quick to load. The site is equipped with an internal search engine, which is a good thing given its size. The graphical navigation menu (which helps you maneuver throughout the Web site) found at the bottom of some of its pages is cryptic however; the newer version appears to be more informative.

Title (or descriptor):	American Medical Informatics Association
Owner:	American Medical Informatics Association (AMIA)
URL (Web address):	`http://www.amia.org/`
Rating:	★★★

Much improved over the years, the AMIA Web site offers users information about technology in healthcare. The home page is divided into six distinct categories, including meetings and educational events, membership and services, publications, the organization's structure and operations, additional information about informatics, and background information about previous AMIA meetings. Complete abstracts are available on this site from the AMIA journal, *Journal of the American Medical Informatics Association*, dating back to 1994. A simple site, but full of useful information helpful in keeping on top of the medical informatics field.

 American Psychiatric Association

Title (or descriptor):	American Psychiatric Association
Owner:	American Psychiatric Association
URL (Web address):	http://www.psych.org/
Rating:	★★★★

The Web site of the APA is so large and layered that if it didn't have its own internal search engine you might spend days trying to get to the actual abundance of information. The site is filled with a wide variety of information on mental disorders, on the professional association itself, consumer-oriented "Let's Talk Facts" brochures, and a whole lot more for psychiatrists and laypeople. It is relatively well-designed with sharp graphics. The Web site is, however, much too hierarchical in its information presentation, requiring the reader to access submenu after submenu to get to the useful content. The graphics tend to be overdone as well, and there are far too many of them. The font size used throughout the site is *large* and easy to read.

Professional information on the site includes a section for APA members, ethics, a catalog of current offerings, information on the annual Psychiatric Institute and APA convention, a number of publications, and additional links. The catalog offers links to information on APA Periodicals (*American Journal of Psychiatry, Psychiatric Services,* and *Psychiatric News*), publications ("DSM-IV & Related Products," "Practice Guidelines," "Task Force Reports," and "Ethics Booklets"), multimedia products, educational programs and seminars, a job bank, and information on their insurance and consultation services. But the majority of information on the APA site appears to consist of educational brochures and similar information on mental disorders. This includes well-written and lengthy articles on depression, anxiety, eating disorders, coping with HIV and AIDS, and substance abuse, among others. Research funding information and training manuals can also be found on the Web site.

Title (or descriptor):	American Psychiatric Nurses Association
Owner:	American Psychiatric Nurses Association (APNA)
URL (Web address):	`http://www.apna.org/`
Rating:	★★

The Web site for the APNA offers the standard organizational fare—membership information, contact information, organizational information, and past tables of contents for its own *Journal of the American Psychiatric Nurses Association*. Graphics are small and quick to load, but are from standard graphic libraries on the Web, making them less than customized or professional. Announcements and links to other related Web sites round out this site.

Title (or descriptor):	American Psychoanalytic Association
Owner:	American Psychoanalytic Association (APsA)
URL (Web address):	`http://www.apsa.org/`
Rating:	★★★

The American Psychoanalytic Association (APsA) has approximately 3,000 individual members and a Web site offering its members a great deal of information. While psychoanalysis has lagged in the United States, it still enjoys a popular worldwide following and is respected in many schools. Highlighted in a recent visit to their Web site was the APsA's annual meeting. Like many organizational sites, this Web site placed too many links to its offerings on its home page. This design blunder makes it difficult for people to reasonably choose from a short list of topics. Once you do choose, though, you will find a wealth of resources at this site, including the unique ability to send e-mail to any member who has registered an e-mail address. An extraordinary feature of this site is a searchable bibliographic database containing over 30,000 references to books, book reviews, and journal articles of a psychoanalytic orientation. It is original contributions to online resources such as this that make the World Wide Web so valuable. Selected full-text articles from *The American Psychoanalyst* are also available, but they may be slow to update those. Overall, this is a strong Web site and a valuable resource to anyone interested in psychoanalysis.

Title (or descriptor):	American Psychoanalytic Foundation
Owner:	American Psychoanalytic Foundation
URL (Web address):	http://www.cyberpsych.org/apf/
Rating:	★★★

With a simple, clean interface, the American Psychoanalytic Foundation's Web site functions as an effective educational tool and resource for its members and the public interested in learning more about psychoanalysis, Freud's primary psychotherapy method. It appears to be updated on a fairly regular basis and offers information about its programs and projects, recommended reading, upcoming events, and other psychoanalytic news of interest. Strangely absent from the site is information on how to join and become a member of the foundation.

Title (or descriptor):	American Psychological Association
Owner:	American Psychological Association
URL (Web address):	http://www.apa.org/
Rating:	★★★★

A Web site full of useful information about journals as well as consumer information, press releases, and professional information related to the psychological profession. It also serves as an online publishing "mirror" for the psychologist's monthly newspaper, the APA *Monitor*, offering listings from their events and continuing education calendar, classified ads, and select full-text articles every month (http://www.apa.org/monitor/). Design suffers from a lack of overall organization and style standards from page to page within the site, although this continues to improve.

The APA (with over 150,000 psychologist members) rivals the American Psychiatric Association's Web site in its breadth and depth of content. Organized around a somewhat similar hierarchical approach, the site is most effective in providing online material published in traditional media. It offers information for professionals ranging from the full text of the APA's "Ethical Principles and Guidelines" to newsletters (*Practitioner Update* and *Practitioner Focus*, for instance, although neither was up-to-date). The science section provides resources on the directorate's programs and general information, annual report, the "APA Task Force on Intelligence Releases Report," APA science advocacy, awards and funding programs, testing and assessment information, and various psychological science resources online and in the real world. The site gets low marks for not linking to related content on the Web, as most other organizations do.

The Members Services area will be of special value to APA members, as it gives them access to additional services, such as PsychINFO. Members could also search the APA's book and journal offerings and use a professional version of their PsycCrawler Web search engine.

Title (or descriptor):	American Psychological Society
Owner:	American Psychological Society and Hanover College
URL (Web address):	`http://www.psychologicalscience.org/`
Rating:	★★★

The American Psychological Society (APS) Web site, maintained by John Krantz at Hanover College, is a cornucopia of online professional resources. Although I don't much care for the home page (which is *way* too confusing!), you will find employment listings, information about the society, federal funding updates, annual convention information, and much more. Many of the past issues of the *APS Observer* can also be found here, as well as past APS convention proceedings. The graphical buttons are a bit outdated, and some information does not appear to be updated regularly. This site is also home to many additional Internet resources of use to professionals. These include links to hundreds of psychology department Web sites throughout the world and a large listing of journal Web sites. Links are arranged by categories: teaching, research, mental health, employment, graduate student, and a host of other resources. Some areas, such as the "Teaching Resources" section, are very well done and offer a lot of topics not found anywhere else online today. The site is about average to navigate around in, but the breadth of content offered more than makes up for its navigational and design shortcomings.

Title (or descriptor):	Association for the Advancement of Gestalt Therapy
Owner:	Association for the Advancement of Gestalt Therapy (AAGT)
URL (Web address):	`http://www.aagt.org/`
Rating:	★★

The Association for the Advancement of Gestalt Therapy (AAGT) site explains the basics about the Association, including an introduction to the AAGT, a description of the special interest groups in the organization, information about their annual international conference, a simplified summary of Gestalt therapy, a listing of Gestalt, psychology, and psychotherapy online resources, and a short glossary of Gestalt terminology. I wish more time was spent expanding the Gestalt area and information sections, rather than adding links to other pages. Membership information (including the organization's bylaws) is available. It's a solid Web site with potential.

Title (or descriptor):	Association for Applied Psychophysiology and Biofeedback
Owner:	Association for Applied Psychophysiology and Biofeedback (AAPB)
URL (Web address):	http://www.aapb.org/
Rating:	★★★

This association represents clinicians who are interested in psychophysiology or biofeedback. A well-constructed site offers links to their mission statement, membership information, research, FAQ about biofeedback, conference listings, and links to other sites. Current news and events round out this attractive site.

Title (or descriptor):	The Association of Black Psychologists
Owner:	The Association of Black Psychologists
URL (Web address):	http://www.abpsi.org/
Rating:	★★★

Much improved since its inception, the Association for Black Psychologists' Web site now offers extensive information about this organization. This information includes the organization's history and vision, contact and membership information, and publications of interest.

Title (or descriptor):	Association for the Scientific Study of Consciousness
Owner:	Association for the Scientific Study of Consciousness (ASSC)
URL (Web address):	http://assc.caltech.edu/
Rating:	★★★

The Association for the Scientific Study of Consciousness (ASSC) states on their Web site that the association

> promotes research within cognitive science, neuroscience, philosophy, and other relevant disciplines in the sciences and humanities, directed toward understanding the nature, function, and underlying mechanisms of consciousness.

The Web site offers additional information about the organization, its bylaws, how to join as a member, and journal information. ASSC is the sponsor of the online refereed electronic journal, *PSYCHE*, as well as the regular print journal, *Consciousness and Cognition*; information about these journals and how to subscribe to them is available here.

The real depth of content at this site lies in its very extensive bibliography, put together by Thomas Metzinger and David Chalmers. This selected bibliography covers books and articles on consciousness in philosophy, cognitive science, and neuroscience since 1970. It consists of three main sections: monographs, edited collections of papers, and articles, and it is completely searchable. It is constantly updated on the Web site and is an invaluable addition to the online world.

Title (or descriptor):	Canadian Psychological Association
Owner:	Canadian Psychological Association
URL (Web address):	`http://www.cpa.ca/`
Rating:	★★★

The Canadian Psychological Association (CPA) Web site is a good example of an online resource with a lot of information, as well as a lot of potential. Attractively designed and well-organized, the CPA offers a wealth of background and history about the organization, a listing of staff should you wish to contact the CPA, an online searchable membership directory, and a few publications. The publications include the *Canadian Journal of Behavioural Science* as well as the CPA's official quarterly newspaper, *Psynopsis*. I was disappointed to see that although the journal offered full-text articles all the way back to 1992, the most recent issues hadn't been updated for over 8 months. Since placing full-text articles on their Web site apparently was a project of some kind, it may be that the project is over, and new articles will never be published online. Progress reports were supposed to be published quarterly, but I could only find two out of four quarters. After reading through a half-dozen files on the project, I still wasn't clear as to its outcome. Noticeably lacking on the CPA Web site are any

ONLINE DOESN'T ALWAYS MEAN ON TIME

One of the most frustrating aspects of surfing the Web and looking for online information is determining how often a publisher or organization decides to place their real-world print articles on their Web site. A lot of sites place articles online without carefully deciding on a schedule for updates or further publication and without assigning the appropriate staff for this online responsibility. This short-sightedness is common among Web developers. They understand that content is important and rush to place as much of it as possible online when they first develop their Web site. But as the weeks turn into months, the one person responsible for maintaining up-to-date content often turns to other tasks or responsibilities. Before anyone realizes, the site has become woefully outdated in a matter of months.

Some sites have developed a sensible and well-conceived publishing policy ahead of time. The American Psychological Association's *Monitor* (`http://www.apa.org/monitor/`), CME's *Psychiatric Times* (`http://www.psychiatrictimes.com/about.html`), and the American Psychiatric Association's *Psychiatric News* (`http://pn.psychiatryonline.org/`) have all developed online publication procedures that make them reliable and useful to readers. Sometimes, the online version appears before the print publication is available! A Web site does not have to offer its entire real-world print offerings online to be successful; they simply need to let their readers know what they do offer online and how often they make new items available.

resources or information about mental disorders for either laypeople or professionals. Their general links to other psychology Web sites is eclectic and missing a lot of popular and useful sites commonly found on other lists. Available in English and French versions.

Title (or descriptor):   Cape Cod Institute
Owner: Cape Cod Institute
URL (Web address):   `http://www.cape.org/`
Rating: ★★★

The Cape Cod Institute offers symposia every summer for keeping mental health professionals up-to-date on the latest developments in psychology, treatment, psychiatry, and mental health. Renowned professionals often speak at this institute because it is a relaxed environment and allows greater interaction between faculty and participants. The Web site gracefully outlines the available workshops and offers much information about lodging and the like to potential participants. An interactive, Web-based discussion forum is even offered to allow participants to chat with one another about past and future courses.

Title (or descriptor):	Clinical Social Work Federation
Owner:	Clinical Social Work Federation (CSWF)
URL (Web address):	`http://www.cswf.org/`
Rating:	★★★★

The number and degree of good social work resources online is not at all large. This site goes a long way to correct that problem, in providing a central resource for clinical social workers. Its resources include information about the federation, a conference and workshop calendar, information on how to subscribe to a number of social worker mailing lists, legislative and news updates, links to state agencies and social work societies, as well as a number of publications including *The Family Therapy Practice Academy News Notes*. The site is generally well organized and information is presented in an easy-to-read manner.

Title (or descriptor):	The Industrial–Organizational Psychologist
Owner:	Society for Industrial and Organizational Psychology (SIOP)
URL (Web address):	`http://www.siop.org/`
Rating:	★★★

Home to *The Industrial–Organizational Psychologist* newsletter, the official publication of the Society for Industrial and Organizational Psychology (SIOP), this Web site has a lot of links and resources. Back issues and complete articles of the newsletter are available on the site, dating back to 1995. The site has grown in content and professionalism over the years. In addition to the newsletter, the site hosts an e-mail directory of SIOP members, organizational, membership, conference, and contact information, and postion papers adopted by SIOP. A call for proposals for its annual conference, information on how to order audio cassettes from its last conference, and available postions and internships are also included in this continuously-updated and growing site. Links to related I-O Web sites, grant searches, and discussion forums round out this site.

Title (or descriptor):	International Society for Mental Health Online
Owner:	International Society for Mental Health Online
URL (Web address):	http://www.ismho.org/
Rating:	★★★

Please see the full description of this professional association in Chapter 11.

Title (or descriptor):	National Association of Cognitive-Behavioral Therapists
Owner:	National Association of Cognitive-Behavioral Therapists (NACBT)
URL (Web address):	http://www.nacbt.org/
Rating:	★★

A site that is apparently still under construction (many of its links don't work), it provides information about the National Association of Cognitive-Behavioral Therapists (NACBT). It is devoted to the teaching and practice of cognitive-behavioral psychotherapy. A membership form, basic information about the association and its leadership, and contact information is available from the content-slim site.

Title (or descriptor):	National Association of School Psychologists
Owner:	National Association of School Psychologists (NASP)
URL (Web address):	http://www.nasponline.org/
Rating:	★★

The Association represents the interests of school psychologists to advance children's mental health and educational competence. Its Web site is fairly large and up to date, but relies on dynamic menus that pop up as you scroll your mouse pointer over options such as Members, Conventions, Publications, Advocacy, and the like. Using such a menu system on sites has become increasingly frequent, yet their usability remains low because the options available under each section are hidden until you uncover them manually. The submenus will also be difficult for those with less-than-perfect eyesight in reading the small print. Clicking on your Web browser's "Back" button will not always return you to the previous page because of the way the site was designed. To their credit, however, the NASP does provide a handi-capped accessible, plain-text home page. Despite these challenges in usability, the site provides a wealth of information about the organization, including a search engine that allowed me to find more specific information. A public membership directory was not apparent.

Title (or descriptor):	National Association of Social Workers
Owner:	National Association of Social Workers (NASW)
URL (Web address):	`http://www.socialworkers.org/`
Rating:	★★★

Having grown and added extensively to their Web site in the past year, the National Association of Social Workers now has a great resource online. While the home page offers too many and sometimes repetitive choices, the site is generally well-designed and easy to navigate. The site is divided into a number of major catagories, includ-ing organizational, contact, and membership information, a "what's new" section, a jobs listing, insurance trust, publications index, ethical code of conduct, advocacy work, social work practice, NASW credentials, latest press releases and news from NASW, and links to related Web resources. In addition to this information, the site has a Clinical Register Online. This database allows a user to search for a clinical so-cial worker within their community. It worked as expected when I tried it and quickly located 28 clinical social workers within the Columbus, Ohio area. The site sometimes loses its lower navigation bar when browsing certain areas (such as the Clinical Register Online or the NASW Press area). A listing of related meetings and calls for papers fills out an excellent online social work resource.

Title (or descriptor):	Society for the Exploration of Psychotherapy Integration
Owner:	Society for the Exploration of Psychotherapy Integration
URL (Web address):	`http://www.cyberpsych.org/sepi/`
Rating:	★★

The society is an "interdisciplinary organization of professionals interested in ap-proaches to psychotherapy that are not limited by a single orientation," according to its Web site. Irregularly maintained, the site is a simple affair that links to some articles published by its members, and other organizations or Web sites of interest.

Title (or descriptor):	Society for Neuronal Regulation
Owner:	Society for Neuronal Regulation
URL (Web address):	`http://www.snr-jnt.org/`
Rating:	★★★

A site that will mainly interest professionals in neurofeedback, such as EEG or biofeedback. Its main offerings are full-length articles as well as abstracts reprinted with permission from their own members, as well as some reprinted from regular professional journals. This site is updated irregularly and only a few links to other pages may be found here.

Title (or descriptor):	Society for the Psychology of Women
Owner:	Division 35, American Psychological Association
URL (Web address):	`http://www.apa.org/divisions/div35/`
Rating:	★★★

The Society for the Psychology of Women was established in 1973 as Division 35 of the American Psychological Association, but anyone can join as a member. The society is devoted to providing an organization for anyone interested in teaching, research, or practice in the psychology of women. The group's purpose is to promote feminist scholarship and practice and to advocate action toward public policies that advance equality and social justice.

Title (or descriptor):	Teachers of Psychology in Secondary Schools (TOPSS)
Owner:	American Psychological Association
URL (Web address):	`http://www.apa.org/ed/topss/`
Rating:	★★★

The Teachers of Psychology in Secondary Schools organization is interested in helping promote the introduction of students to psychology in high school through curriculum suggestions, essay contents, and teacher workshops. Information about the organization may be found here, as well as specific unit plans for teachers on a variety of psychology subjects (e.g., personality, biological bases of behavior, statistics). A well-organized site with a wealth of information for psychology teachers.

Title (or descriptor):	World Health Organization
Owner:	World Health Organization
URL (Web address):	http://www.who.org/
Rating:	★★★

Certainly an international organization the size and scope of the World Health Organization (WHO) should offer a Web site equally large. WHO doesn't fail to deliver on its Web presence, offering readers a large site full of background and history of the organization, descriptions and information on its multitude of programs administered throughout the world, and a large archive of statements published by the organization on international medical and health issues and crises. Statistical information in the form of the *Weekly Epidemiological Record* (WER) and the *Statistical Information System* (WHOSIS) is available through the Web site, as is a complete list of WHO publications and database offerings. Readers may also find press releases, contact information, online newsletters (although how up-to-date they are varies widely), and the *World Health Report*, published annually. Some files are in the "portable document format" (PDF), which requires the Adobe Acrobat reader. The Web site itself is well designed and offers an internal search engine.

HOW CAN I FIND THE ADDRESS OR PHONE NUMBER OF MY STATE PROFESSIONAL ASSOCIATION?

While there is no central organizational listing online for professional associations at the state or local level, you may find them through a number of common methods. The first place to check is with the national organization's Web site. For example, a listing of contact information for state associations of psychologists is available on the American Psychological Association's Web site (http://www.apa.org/practice/refer.html). Such a list will often indicate whether a state association has a Web site (and provide an appropriate link). Division information is also available. Psychologists, for instance, will find complete division information (including contacts, addresses, Web sites, and e-mail addresses) on the American

Psychological Association Web site (`http://www.apa.org/`); psychiatrists will find similar types of information on the American Psychiatric Association's Web site (`http://www.psych.org/`).

You can also check one of the Web sites that specializes in this kind of information or a subject guide. For example, Myron Pulier, MD offers a listing of over 1,400 mental health organizations around the world (`http://www.umdnj.edu/psyevnts/psyjumps.html#Meetings`).

In many cases, at this time at least, obtaining information about state and local chapters of professional associations or related organizations can only be obtained by making a telephone call. Any agency or organization directly related to the government, however, might be found on your local state government's home page. For a listing of where your local government's Web site is located, check Yahoo!'s index of U.S. states (`http://www.yahoo.com/Government/`).

HOW DO I GET INVOLVED IN COMBATING THE SOCIAL STIGMATIZATION OF MENTAL DISORDERS?

There are many national and international organizations whose sole purpose is to educate the public and reduce the stigmatization of mental disorders. Nowhere are such advocates more vocal than in the online world, where an individual can reach thousands of people with very little effort and at almost no cost. Naturally professional associations such as the American Psychological Association (`http://www.apa.org/`) and the American Psychiatric Association (`http://www.psych.org/`) have taken leadership roles in this effort. On each of their Web sites, you will find specific areas devoted to publicizing what is currently known about mental disorders to the public and media. Certainly these sites are a good place to find such information and get started in becoming more actively involved in promoting mental health issues online.

The quality and bias of the information is determined by the organization publishing it, just as it is in the real world. With that caveat in mind, I will now discuss a few other organizations, in the real world as well as online, whose sole goal is to promote the dissemination of information about mental disorders and to help educate the public about proper and effective treatment options. These organizations usually go beyond simply present-ing information and allowing consumers and laypeople to form their own opinions. Often they are promoting a particular viewpoint, which may or may not be validated by current research. Many professionals are involved within these organizations, however, and their online efforts reflect their commitment to their cause.

Title (or descriptor):	NAMI New York City Metro
Owner:	Alliance for the Mentally Ill
URL (Web address):	`http://www.nami-nyc-metro.org/`
Rating:	★★★

The Web site, maintained by NAMI New York City Metro, has a great deal of useful information on mental disorders, reducing the stigmatization of them in our society today, and how you can become more active in mental health advocacy in your local community. As one of the largest chapters of the National Alliance for the Mentally Ill, NAMI/NYC adopts the same philosophical stance on mental disorders being "neurobiological disorders (NBDs)." They heavily emphasize neurochemical inter-ventions and radical treatments such as electroconvulsive therapy (ECT). Both NAMI/NYC (as well as NAMI) were set up to help support family members and in-dividuals who suffer from mental disorders. They also support education to the so-ciety at large about these disorders. Addressing a common misunderstanding that people with mental disorders are somehow morally weak, these organizations have become recognized authorities for their advocacy and education efforts on behalf of the mentally ill.

NAMI/NYC's Web site reflects the organization's goals by offering information about their mission, policies, meetings, local resources, and support groups. Updated news keeps readers informed about events of interest in mental health and the com-munity. The site also features an "Ask the Doctor" section that allows users to ask a medical question of a physician. The site appears to be regularly updated, is simply designed, and loads quickly.

Title (or descriptor):	National Alliance for the Mentally Ill (NAMI)
Owner:	National Alliance for the Mentally Ill

URL (Web address):   `http://www.nami.org/`

Rating: ★★★

The National Alliance for the Mentally Ill (NAMI) follows much the same philosophical guidelines as outlined in the NAMI/NYC review. On their home page, under "About Mental Illness," NAMI states, "Mental illnesses are biologically-based brain disorders . . . " It is precisely because of this type of misinformation that NAMI is sometimes controversial and doesn't count an abundance of nonmedical mental health professionals and psychologists among its ranks.

NAMI's Web site *is* full of generally useful information and articles on mental disorders, although biased toward a medical model and, hence, medical treatment. Readers will find membership and NAMI conference information, as well as articles on a number of disorders such as schizophrenia, bipolar disorder, major depression, obsessive–compulsive disorders, and "neurobiological brain disorders" in general. The articles are oriented toward laypeople and contain little detailed information (except when discussing medications). The research findings (which highlight only medical research, not social science research) are also irregularly updated.

The site itself is quick to load, and its latest design makes it easier to find information oriented toward different populations (researchers, consumers, advocates, etc.).

Title (or descriptor):   National Mental Health Association (NMHA)

Owner: National Mental Health Association

URL (Web address):   `http://www.nmha.org/`

Rating: ★★★

Probably the best and by far the most balanced organization devoted to mental health advocacy and education efforts, the National Mental Health Association (NMHA) offers an educational site. According to the NMHA, they are "the nation's only citizen volunteer advocacy organization dedicated to addressing all aspects of mental health and mental illnesses."

Their Web site is full of useful and relevant information on mental disorders and treatment (under the "Information" category), as well as resources on public policy and legislative alerts (under "Advocacy"), news releases, and prevention information. It is updated regularly so the news and legislative alerts are usually fresh. The organization also does a good job with providing two real-world publications for reading on their Web site, the quarterly *NMHA Prevention Update* and *The Bell*. The site is well designed with attractive but minimal graphics.

Title (or descriptor):	Support Coalition International
Owner:	Support Coalition International
URL (Web address):	http://www.mindfreedom.org/
Rating:	★

At the other end of the spectrum from AMI/FAMI/NAMI is Support Coalition. This organization is against nonconsensual psychiatric treatment, as well as certain forms of treatment, such as electroconvulsive therapy (ECT). Their redesigned Web site makes it easier to find resources and navigate. It offers only tidbits of information supporting their viewpoint and does no better job of presenting an accurate portrayal of our current state of knowledge of mental disorders. About the only useful thing this site *does* offer is information on the pitfalls of ECT, as well as additional information about how to join Support Coalition. Virtually no real-world contact information could be culled from this site, even though they claim to be an independent nonprofit federation of nearly 100 grassroots groups in 13 countries (although none were listed). The information offered is sensationalized, with overuse of exclamation points and large fonts.

Book Publishers, Bookstores, and Journals Online

Numerous book publishers, bookstores, and journals are online and can be easily found—if you know where to look. Most book publishers provide some type of searchable online database of their current offerings, as do the online bookstores. Book publishers also offer contact information for ordering a book, a catalog, or to request further print information about something they publish. Bookstores online allow you to purchase books right from your computer with a credit card or by calling a toll-free number. Some bookstores even offer a discount up to 30% for some books and 10% for most others. What is nicest about online bookstores is the ability to enter keywords or search terms into their database search engine to locate books on a certain topic or with a certain word in their title. Potentially, this can allow you to locate, on your own, even obscure books on any particular subject. Try that at your local bookstore! Typically, journal Web sites offer you the ability to catch up with a print journal's current table of contents and read subscription information. Other journals may offer the complete text of articles online. Some journals are published *only* online, allowing you to read full-text, professional articles at no charge.

WHERE CAN I GO TO FIND BOOK PUBLISHERS AND INFORMATION ABOUT THE BOOKS THEY PUBLISH?

Nearly every book publisher has joined the age of technology and moved onto the World Wide Web. The quality of the Web sites vary greatly, as does the amount of interactivity offered (e.g., the ability to buy a book from them). Most offer a basic corporate Web site, with information about the publishing company, its corporate makeup and officers, contact information, and the like. Additionally some offer access to their publishing database, so you can hunt down titles and authors, and even find out if the book is still in print. What follows is an abbreviated listing of some of the larger mental health professional publishers. A more extensive listing of mainstream publishers is available from Yahoo! (`http://dir.yahoo.com/Business_and_Economy/Shopping_ and_Services/Publishers/`), the Open Directory Project (`http:// dmoz.org/Business/Publishing_and_Printing/Publishers/`), or AcqWeb (`http://acqweb.library.vanderbilt.edu/`).

Title (or descriptor):	Academic Press
Owner:	Elsevier Science
URL (Web address):	`http://www.apcatalog.com/`
Rating:	★★

A searchable database makes finding a book from this publisher quick and easy. Both simple keyword searches and advanced searches are available. Their database contains over 6,000 titles. Since being acquired by Elsevier Science, Academic Press's Web site has become a part of the larger corporate parent's site. This has made for a less pleasant book-browsing experience, with many pages often including awkward and lengthy column lists of subjects or books.

Title (or descriptor):   American Psychiatric Press

Owner: American Psychiatric Press, Inc.

URL (Web address):   http://www.appi.org/

Rating: ★★

Featured titles grace the home page of the American Psychiatric Press Web site. The site includes information and some descriptions on books, journals, and multimedia products. Listings of offerings are arranged by author or subject, and descriptions were often lacking. The Web site performed very slowly at the times I visited it, and the ordering process was clunky.

Title (or descriptor):   American Psychological Association Press

Owner: American Psychological Association

URL (Web address):   http://www.apa.org/books/

URL (Web address):   http://www.apa.org/journals/

Rating: ★★★

Descriptions of books and journals published by the American Psychological Association (APA) may be found on this Web site under two separate categories. The search engine works but provides cryptic results. In the books area, the "Recent Releases" category is updated monthly. Books listed under subject categories (Education Books, Scientific Books, Practice Related Books, etc.) are arranged alphabetically. You can print out an order form, but can't order online. A large, complete site for information on any publication from the APA.

Title (or descriptor):   Classics in the History of Psychology

Owner: Christopher Green

URL (Web address):   http://psychclassics.yorku.ca/

Rating: ★★★★

Although not a publisher in the traditional sense, Christopher Green has collected and indexed hundreds of classic books and articles that are no longer copyrighted.

The collection is searchable or available to browse by topic or author's name. The articles and books are available for free, in their entirety, on the site itself. An amazing historical collection of psychology texts that is well organized and updated regularly.

Title (or descriptor):	Guilford Press
Owner:	Guilford Press
URL (Web address):	`http://www.guilford.com/`
Rating:	★★★

Information on every Guilford publication is readily accessible, either by searching for an author/editor, title, or keyword using their search engine, or by browsing a list of titles, which is organized by subject area. Graphics are professional and the site is well organized, with contact information for Guilford at the bottom of every page. Guilford is the publisher of this book. Guilford also makes excerpts available from selected books, making it easier to decide whether or not to purchase a given volume. This is a nice touch not yet found on many publishers' Web sites.

Title (or descriptor):	MIT Press
Owner:	MIT Press
URL (Web address):	`http://www-mitpress.mit.edu/`
Rating:	★★★

You may use either their search engine (which is more complicated than necessary) or browse through their indices of books categorized by topic to find a title published from 1993 to 1997.

Title (or descriptor):	W. W. Norton & Company
Owner:	W. W. Norton & Company
URL (Web address):	`http://www.wwnorton.com/`
Rating:	★★

A graphics-intensive home page takes a while to load and offers a confusing array of choices. You can browse their catalog and search it.

Title (or descriptor):	Oxford University Press
Owner:	Oxford University Press USA
URL (Web address):	`http://www.oup-usa.org/`
Rating:	★★★

You may search or browse through their book catalog. A large home page graphic will take a while to load on most people's browsers.

Title (or descriptor):	Prentice Hall Publishing
Owner:	Prentice Hall Publishing
URL (Web address):	`http://www.prenhall.com/`
Rating:	★★★

By choosing the "Humanities and Social Sciences" division on Prentice Hall's home page, you can browse by book title through the "Course Catalog" option. Choosing "Custom Catalog" gives you a search form in which to enter a query. Book information includes a description, table of contents, and ordering information. The site is large and attractively designed.

Title (or descriptor):	Princeton University Press
Owner:	Princeton University Press
URL (Web address):	`http://www.pupress.princeton.edu/`
Rating:	★★★

A large home page graphic (which appears to be common among book publishers!) detracts from an otherwise excellent and solid site. Both searching and browsing of their catalog is available, as is a list of out-of-print titles (which is handy).

Title (or descriptor):	Sage Publications
Owner:	Sage Publications
URL (Web address):	`http://www.sagepub.com/`
Rating:	★★

Sage has redesigned their Web site in recent years and now features a more standard and easy-to-navigate site that makes browsing or searching for books on specific topics or titles easy. The site feels more like a store with a generic inventory, however, than a book publisher. Many book covers' graphics are not available, and information on a specific title tends to be too brief to make a purchase decision.

Title (or descriptor):	John Wiley & Sons, Inc., Publishers
Owner:	John Wiley & Sons, Inc., Publishers
URL (Web address):	`http://www.wiley.com/`
Rating:	★★★

Offering a large and somewhat difficult-to-navigate Web site, John Wiley & Sons' online catalogs vary in quality. For instance, most of the journals listed have their own Web pages, with lengthy descriptions, editorial board listings, notes for contributors, and subscription information. Books, on the other hand, often are lacking any descriptive information. Numerous broken links were discovered. You may browse through titles or use their search engine (which was also broken when I tried using it).

WHERE DO I GO TO BUY A BOOK ONLINE?

What's nice about the online world today is the ability to shop at your convenience and in the privacy of your home or office. Book buying is ideally suited to the online world. Especially useful is the ability to find and order used or out-of-print books through some online bookstores. Although there is no central location online to find a listing of all the online bookstores as of this writing, you can find a pretty good list of them at the Open Directory Project (`http://dmoz.org/Shopping/Publications/Books/`).

Some people have Web sites today that link to specific book titles in one of the bookstores listed below and call it a "bookstore." These are not real online bookstores because they do not do any of the actual selling or shipping of books—they are just making recommendations for purchase (much like the *New York Review of Books* does). The owners of such sites usually get a referral fee for every book a user from their site buys at the online bookstore, so it is an incentive for them to list as many books as possible on their site. These sites may provide some type of additional benefit through their book reviews, but reviews can also be found directly at the bookstores themselves (such as Amazon.com). Review quality itself can vary greatly— even on the bookstore sites—and the reviewers' background is rarely available. Bookstore sites, however, allow ordinary users to rate the quality of review, so that future readers of the review might have some additional guideline on which to base their weight of the review. These types of book review Web sites, of which there are many, are not reviewed or recommended in this section.

amazon.com.

Title (or descriptor):	Amazon.com
Owner:	Amazon.com
URL (Web address):	`http://www.amazon.com/`
Rating:	★★★★

Amazon.com offers nearly every book published by anyone through their database and ordering system online. Since they don't actually have to warehouse every title, they can stack the virtual shelves as high as they'd like! They've done exactly that, listing millions of titles within their extensive database. Naturally they don't actually have *every* in-print book available for immediate shipment. But for most popular, mainstream books, they offer quick delivery times and easy online ordering. A "Special Order" notation next to many of their professional titles means the book may take 4 to 6 weeks to receive. Amazon.com also offers users the ability to search for used, hard-to-find, and out-of-print items. Each book listing includes the availability of the book (most are shipped within 2 to 3 days), publisher, author(s), publication date, binding (hardcover or paperback), and number of pages. Most books are available at a discounted retail price. Ordering can be conducted through a secure online transaction server (where it is safe to enter in credit card information and transmit it over the Internet) or through a toll-free phone number.

Searching through the Amazon.com database is preferable to browsing, although a browsing option is available. Using one of their many search engines (keyword, title, author, subject, advanced), users can enter in any terms or part of a term they are searching on. The only drawback to a database so large is that it is generally geared more toward popular books, not professional titles. So some professional titles may not be available within 2 to 3 days, and they will usually not be offered at any discount. As with any search engine, you should read their "Search Tips" to get the most from your queries. Amazon.com has expanded far beyond its original bookstore model, and now offers one-stop shopping for books, videos, music, toys, electronics, auctions, and more. They don't do as good a job in these additional areas, and often their prices are higher than other Web sites that specialize in them.

Title (or descriptor):	Barnes & Noble
Owner:	Barnes & Noble
URL (Web address):	`http://www.bn.com/`
Rating:	★★★

Barnes & Noble came to the game of online book selling later than Amazon.com, and so had a fair amount of catching up to do. Despite having a recognizable real-world brand name, and brick-and-mortar stores to back it up, the Barnes & Noble site doesn't leverage either very well. Barnes & Noble seems to have duplicated key aspects of the Amazon.com model of success, from low prices, a selection covering millions of books, and allowing people to enter their own review of books, right down to navigational tabs to move from section to section on the site. The resemblance and feature-match is perhaps just a bit too canny and unoriginal. Originality would be allowing a user to order a book through the site and pick it up at one of their local bookstores, a feature Amazon.com couldn't easily match. Nothing like that exists on the site today, though.

But competition is good for you, the consumer. If Amazon.com can't deliver a book you need at the time and price desired, visit Barnes & Noble's site.

ABOUT PRINT AND ELECTRONIC JOURNALS

With all of the benefits of online technology at your fingertips, it makes sense that publishing research in a more timely manner is in the front of many professionals' minds. With traditional peer-reviewed print journals, going from submission to final publication of a research study can take years for some journals, and many months for others. Imagine what could be done by removing the lengthy print publishing step and replacing it with a streamlined online process.

There are two types of journal Web sites found online: print journals with a Web site and electronic journals that have no print counterpart. The former is far more common than the latter. Print journals will publish a Web page to offer information about the journal and how to subscribe to it. They may also publish the current table of contents as a service to online readers and potential subscribers. Some publishers take this a step further and also publish abstracts of recent or current articles. Finally, some "go all the way" and make the full text of one or two of their current articles available on their Web site. Additionally, some journals also offer the option of reading or searching full-text articles online if you are already a subscriber to the print-version of the journal. Remember, if you're looking for information on how to search the journal articles themselves, please refer to Chapter 7.

The second type of Web site is one on which the journal is published exclusively online. These journals were originally experiments in electronic publishing, such as the American Psychological Association's sponsorship of *Pycoloquy*. They have quickly caught on with online readers, though, because they are available without charge and offer refreshing content online (which is all too often lacking in print journals). If online publishing of your own work is an intriguing concept to you, you'll find more information about it at the end of this chapter.

WHERE CAN I GO TO FIND BOTH PRINT JOURNALS AND ONLINE JOURNALS (E-JOURNALS) IN MY FIELD?

The first step to finding online, refereed, professional journals devoted to the kind of topics you're interested in is to look in one of the large journal indices, referred to as "guides" below. They all include some descriptive information about the journal's Web site. This information usually includes the journal's title, and a brief description of the journal.

Some guides list how much information a print journal hosts on its Web site. It is most common to find a print journal's current (and sometimes, past) tables of contents online. This may be helpful in browsing journal titles that interest you to see whether any articles in that issue may be worth reading. It is less common to find abstracts from current and past issues, and least common is to find the actual full text of the articles themselves. All the guides listed below index both electronic journals as well as print journals. Some guides may also include links to professional papers that may not have ever appeared in regular print journals, conference proceedings, and bibliographies.

Guides to Journals and Professional Articles

Title (or descriptor):	Electronic Journals and Periodicals
Owner:	Hanover College Psychology Department
URL (Web address):	

`http://psych.hanover.edu/Krantz/journal.html`

Rating: ★★★

This is one of the older and smaller listings of psychology and related journals and periodicals online. It is still regularly updated and organized alphabetically. Other listings include all the journals found here, but this is a good place to stop by if you're already on the Web or can use a quicker, smaller list of journals. This site also includes listings of some general periodicals that aren't necessarily specific to psychology (e.g., *Academe This Week, Discover Magazine, Electronic Journal on Virtual Culture, Journal of Computer Mediated Communication, Computer-Mediated Communication Magazine, The Journal of NIH Research, Nature Genetics*). It offers some select conference proceedings (e.g., the Sixth and Seventh Annual Convention of the American Psychological Society, 23rd International Conference of Applied Psychology, among others) and has links to one of many MEDLINE search engines available online and a few online bibliographies (*Chinese Psychological Studies, The Drug Discrimination Bibliography, Hong Kong Psychological Studies*). There's really no rhyme or reason to the topics listed here, except that they are available online. This journal listing is compiled and maintained by John H. Krantz, PhD.

Title (or descriptor):	MedWeb: Electronic Newsletters and Journals
Owner:	MedWeb–Emory University Health Sciences Center Library
URL (Web address):	`http://www.medweb.emory.edu/`
Rating:	★★

A very large index of journals and newsletters that have some type of online presence. Although large, the descriptions are less than informative, often involving nothing more than the name of the journal. While a good list to browse for a medically related journal, it is not as helpful or mental health–specific as some other online offerings.

Title (or descriptor): Neurosciences on the Internet
Owner: Neil A. Busis, MD
URL (Web address): http://www.neuroguide.com/
Rating: ★★

This listing consists of journals oriented toward the neurosciences, divided into four categories: (1) journals that offer full-text articles online, (2) journals that offer abstracts online, (3) journals that have only their tables of contents online, and (4) other journals. Dr. Busis also provides a list of other online indices of journals. The lists of journals he provides are lengthy and complete. However, no additional information other than the journal's name is available through this site.

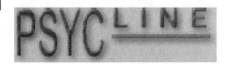

Title (or descriptor): PSYCLINE
Owner: Armin Günther
URL (Web address): http://www.psycline.org/
Rating: ★★★★

Armin Günther has long maintained one of the most comprehensive and up-to-date databases of psychology and social science journals on the Web. This database allows a user to quickly locate a journal's Web site. PSYCLINE's database of more than 2,000 journals is now available on its own well-designed, attractive site, allowing a user to search by keyword, subject, alphabetical order, or by the amount of information the journal has online (for instance, abstracts versus full-text articles). PSYCLINE is a valuable online resource not only because it offers multiple search methods, but also because it is regularly updated. Both e-journals and print journals with Web sites are included in the database. Search results return a description of the journal, the publisher, a link to its Web site, and what types of information you'll find at the journal's Web site (table of contents, abstracts, full-text articles, etc.). PSYCLINE is by far the best and largest specialized journals database online.

Online Journals and Publications

You can keep up with the treatment literature by examining a few regular online journals or professional newspapers every month, or as often as they publish. Just like perusing a regular print journal at home, you can browse through an online counterpart to keep up-to-date on relevant treatment information. I would recommend placing the following publications on your regular reading list.

MONITOR
ON PSYCHOLOGY

Title (or descriptor):	*The Monitor on Psychology*
Owner:	American Psychological Association
URL (Web address):	`http://www.apa.org/monitor/`
Rating:	★★★★

The American Psychological Association publishes its professional newspaper, *The Monitor*, once every month and provides a wide range of selected news stories, articles, editorials, classifieds, and other useful items on its Web site. Articles date back to March, 1995, and more recent editions include the majority of articles listed in the print version of the newspaper. The site's multiple search engines either didn't work or didn't work very well when I finally tracked one down (it didn't return articles in the current issue of *The Monitor* online, for instance). The articles are often relevant and useful to clinicians in general though, and are very good mirrors of their print counterparts.

Title (or descriptor):	*National Psychologist*
Owner:	Ohio Psychology Publications, Inc.
URL (Web address):	`http://www.nationalpsychologist.com/`
Rating:	★★★

A site I designed but no longer have any association with, the *National Psychologist* is an independent bimonthly newspaper that, while focusing on psychology, often has articles of interest for all mental health practitioners. Three articles from each issue are published on its Web site, as well as information on how to subscribe to the print version of the newspaper.

Title (or descriptor):	*PSYCHE: A Journal on Consciousness*
Owner:	Association for the Scientific Study of Consciousness
URL (Web address):	`http://psyche.cs.monash.edu.au/`
Newsgroup:	`sci.psychology.journals.psyche`
Rating:	★★★

PSYCHE is a refereed, electronic journal dedicated to the interdisciplinary exploration of the nature of consciousness and its relationship to the brain. Publishing material from a wide variety of fields including cognitive science, philosophy, psychology, physics, neuroscience, and artificial intelligence. It is available via the Web, a mailing list, or the newsgroup, `sci.psychology.journals.psyche`. Updated regularly.

Title (or descriptor):	*Psychiatric News*
Owner:	American Psychiatric Association
URL (Web address):	`http://pn.psychiatryonline.org/`
Rating:	★★★★

Featuring full text of back issues since March, 1996, this is the official newspaper of the American Psychiatric Association. As such, it is full of informative articles on the latest treatment approaches for practicing psychiatrists. Other mental health professionals can get important treatment information here as well. It is published every other week in print and online. The Web site has become more lean and text based in recent years, and its articles are easy to find.

Title (or descriptor):	*Psychiatric Times*
Owner:	CME, Inc.

URL (Web address):   `http://www.psychiatrictimes.com/`
Rating: ★★★

Another excellent offering in psychiatry, their archive is a little less complete—although it goes back to early 1994. Only select articles are published online from the *Psychiatric Times*, which is published once a month. But that still usually includes anywhere from five to a dozen articles, on a number of topics relevant to all mental health professionals. Arranged by date, author, title, or topic, the online version of this newspaper is easier to search than the APA's *Psychiatric News* and is also less graphics-intensive.

Title (or descriptor): *Psychiatry Online*
Owner: Ben Green, MB, ChB, MRCPsych
URL (Web address):   `http://www.priory.co.uk/psych.htm`
Rating: ★★★

This site is one of the older online psychiatry sites. It has always been somewhat slow to access for North American users because of its location in the U.K. It is chock full of psychiatric and medically oriented professional articles on a wide range of medication and psychopharmacology topics, as well as electroconvulsive therapy (ECT). Some of its articles can be lengthy and sometimes obscure but many are interesting and informative. The site's graphical layout and navigation have always left a lot to be desired, sporting a home page filled with way too many graphics and choices. It is unclear what type of publishing schedule this online journal adheres to, and new articles and updates are sometimes difficult to locate.

Title (or descriptor): *Psychotherapy Networker*
Owner: Psychotherapy Networker, Inc.
URL (Web address):
     `http://www.psychotherapynetworker.org/`
Rating: ★★★

With a brand-new name (it used to be called the *Family Therapy Networker*), the *Psychotherapy Networker* Web site does an excellent job in supporting its print cousin. In addition to offering a general overview of the magazine, the site features links to magazine features and departments, including the Editor's Letter, Case Studies, In Consultation, Tools of the Trade, Networker News, Bookmarks, Screening Room, and Networker Interviews. The selection of articles on the site provides everything from practice tips and tools for practicing therapists to interesting insights for individuals who are just exploring the topic of psychotherapy. There are a variety of discussion groups, on topics such as the current issue of the magazine, the cases posted, and general topical subjects. The Practice Resources section allows visitors to earn continuing education credits, order training tapes and books, and purchase back issues of the magazine. The site also provides subscription information, along with a complete overview of upcoming Networker Symposiums.

Title (or descriptor):	*Psychwatch Newsletter*
Owner:	Psychwatch, Inc.
URL (Web address):	`http://www.psychwatch.com/`
Rating:	★★

Psychwatch sprouted from a simple concept—provide readers quick access to the latest to mental health news online every week. The newsletter does just that, providing subscribers a quick rundown of relevant headlines each week through their Web site, or an e-mailed newsletter. Their site also offers the usual array of links to related professional resources.

Title (or descriptor):	*Psycoloquy*
Owner:	American Psychological Association & various
URL (Web address):	`http://psycprints.ecs.soton.ac.uk/`
Newsgroup:	`sci.psychology.journals.psycoloquy`
Rating:	★★

Psycoloquy started off as a simple psychology newsletter in 1985 and is currently sponsored in part by the American Psychological Association. It does not mirror print journals' traditional publication standards. Each peer-reviewed "issue" is one article, and each volume is largely based on a select number of topic areas. It is rather confusing to read on the Web at the present time, so I recommend that you subscribe to the journal in its mailing list form. It is published sporadically; some months you may receive multiple issues, and other months you will receive nothing. It can also be read via the newsgroup, `sci.psychology.journals.psycoloquy`. Although claiming a large readership, this established and unique journal is still unknown to many professionals online.

Title (or descriptor):	*Self-Help Magazine*
Owner:	Pioneer Development Resources, Inc.
URL (Web address):	http://www.selfhelpmagazine.com/
Rating:	★★★

This general self-help magazine offers online articles on a great deal of topics, ranging from relationships, dreaming, and sex, to posttraumatic strees disorder, eating disorders, and spirituality. Articles tend to be oriented toward consumers and laypeople, so will be of limited value to most professionals. Not every article is dated, which makes it difficult to discern how up-to-date some information may be. Articles are written by a volunteer staff of professionals and published on the Web site as they are written. This group effort shines in the breadth of topics covered and in the Web site's general layout and design. More recently, this online magazine has been struggling to create more of a community for itself, and in doing so, dilutes its identity and purpose. Quirks abound, ranging from a lack of information about the site's advertising policies (advertising on the site sometimes appears unlabeled in the midst of editorial content) to the Web site's privacy statement, which discusses anonymity more than what the company does with the information it collects on its members.

HOW DO I SUBMIT AN ARTICLE TO AN ONLINE JOURNAL?

When NOT to Publish Online

There are some caveats to seeking online publication that you should be aware of. Publication in a peer-reviewed, print journal is the apex of professional accomplishment. Publication on a mailing list is equal to scribbling your study on a piece of paper and tacking it onto the department's bulletin board. Yet many print journals and their editors consider the online publication of an article or study as equivalent to any kind of previous publication. In other words, they won't accept a piece for consideration if it has already been published online in one form or another. Even if you "publish" your article in a mailing list or newsgroup, it may be considered "already published" and will be rejected on those grounds. This becomes of great concern to professionals when they need to list publications on their vitae or justify research expenditures to a department head or grant agency.

There are places online, however, which have the form and function of a print journal transplanted into an electronic version. Some of these online or electronic journals are peer-reviewed and have excellent and respected editorial boards. No matter what the form, an online publication will still garner fewer accolades than its print counterpart. For the most part, professionals tend to recognize by name which print journals have high or low quality. In the online world, though, it is more difficult to evaluate quality and respectability because everything and everyone is new. So authors need to be careful and aware of these issues before deciding to publish online.

What Is Appropriate for Online Publishing?

Sometimes the decision to publish online is an easy one. Studies or articles that have little to no chance of getting published in a print journal are ideal for online publication. These might include well-designed studies with negative results, studies with nonsignificant results but interesting trends, theoretical treatises that span professional disciplines, pilot studies with pilot data, and ideas for studies that cannot be conducted personally. Individuals who have typically been closed off from publishing results in regular print journals (usually anyone who isn't associated with a university) may also turn to an electronic journal for less academic bias.

What Are the Submission Guidelines for Online Publishing?

If you do decide your article or study is appropriate for an online publication, the next step is tailoring it for an online audience. While nearly any article *can* be published, will people actually *read* it? They probably will if you make it readable and keep it short. Every electronic journal will have their own specific publishing and submission guidelines for authors. But I believe the following are good, general points to keep in mind.

- Most people online have short attention spans. Anything over 1,500 words is likely to lose all but the most devoted readers.

- Graphs, charts, and tables should not be too complicated or large.

- Consider breaking longer articles into separate, smaller parts. These may be better published as a series in the journal, if the editors are willing and find the article needs to retain its length to remain valid and useful.

The main point is: Be flexible! Editors of electronic journals appreciate an author's willingness to edit or format an article for better online reading.

Caveats to Readers of Work Published Online

It is important to keep in mind that anyone can put up a home page or Web site nowadays and call it a "journal" or "magazine." Peer review, therefore, is still a worthwhile process and something you should look for in online journals. Another distinguishing feature of serious, professional online journals is that it has been issued an International Standard Serial Number (ISSN) through the Library of Congress or other official agency. This number means that the publication has been registered and suggests it intends to publish indefinitely online. Last, serious online professional journals will note on their masthead real-world contact information, an editorial board of professionals within the journal's field of interest, and have detailed submission guidelines for publication. While these won't guarantee that the journal's actual content will be of high quality, they *are* indicators of professionalism and stability for the online publication.

10

Finding and Downloading Software Online

Software applications (also referred to as "programs") are what allows your computer to do specific tasks. Want to compile statistics for a research study? You'll need a statistical program such as SPPS or SAS. Want to write a letter to a colleague? You'll need a word processing program such as Word or WordPerfect. Want to create your own Web site? You'll need an authoring program such as HomeSite or FrontPage. Want to write clinical or assessment reports in half the time? You'll need to get a clinical report writer or assessment software, which can help you score and even interpret results. As you can probably guess, there are a wide range of reasons you may want or need additional software. People often do much more work than they need to on their computer when others have written software that can help automate repetitive or boring tasks. Just as you can purchase a book online, you can obtain useful, professional software online.

It seems logical that computer software should be available on the Internet, and it is. There are not only a wide range of computer applications in psychology freely available online, but also many general applications as well. Statistical software and applications, which help you score psychological tests (such as the Rorschach or MMPI), are examples of software available for "downloading" (transferring a program to your computer from the Internet). Futhermore, software doesn't have to be about psychology or clinically oriented to be of use to mental health clinicians or researchers. Using the Internet as a telephone is one example where general software can be of invaluable help, reviewed later in this chapter. There are four major types of software available online: shareware (the most common), crippleware, freeware, and demonstration programs.

TYPES OF SOFTWARE AVAILABLE ONLINE

Shareware

Most of the programs discussed below are "shareware" (from the terms "share" and "software"). Its authors allow you to download it to your computer and try it out for free. But if you continue to use it, you are obligated to purchase it for the asking price (often under $50.00). Many full-fledged software applications for your computer can be tried out and purchased in this manner.

Crippleware

Commercial software is also available online. Sometimes referred to as "crippleware" (from the terms "crippled" and "software"), it is software that does not contain all of its usual functionality. For example, you may able to open a file in one of these programs, but you may not be able to save any changes to the file. This allows you to try out the features of the software, but requires you to pay for it if you like it and want to continue using it. After paying for it, you will be given a registration number, which you enter into the program you already have on your computer. This special number then enables those previously crippled functions. Most major applications, such as Microsoft's word processing program, however, are still only available for purchase through a reseller or computer store.

Freeware

Another type of software is "freeware" or "open source." The authors provide it at no cost to the user, and often make the source code available to anyone. But because it is free, it often does not come with support or in-depth documentation to help you out if you have questions. Sometimes you can e-mail the author directly with your questions, but if it is a popular piece of software, you may not receive a reply. (It usually doesn't hurt to try, especially if you have already looked in the "Help" file included with the software, or on the Web site from which you downloaded the software originally.)

When first published, software programs don't always work quite the way the developer intended. They may contain glitches or errors that cause your computer to do unexpected and unintended things. Software developers can fix or update programs, however, quite easily, and these fixes and updates are available online for nearly any piece of software you may have. The fixes are also referred to as "patches," "updates," or "bug fixes." Software that is still in its testing stages (referred to as "beta" software) is also often available for free online. Once it is finished its beta testing, however, the software may expire (stop working) or may become unsupported from the software developer.

Demonstration Programs

The last common type of online software is a demonstration program. Demonstration programs allow you to take a guided tour through a software application that may be too large, complex, or expensive for the software publisher to just give to you to try out on your own. After you are done taking the tour through the software, you may contact the developer for further information or to purchase the complete software package.

I'M LOOKING FOR A PIECE OF PSYCHOLOGY-RELATED SOFTWARE. CAN I FIND IT ONLINE?

Software is not only available online to download directly, but as mentioned above, you can usually try it out and use it for a period of time before deciding whether to purchase it. This is true both for shareware programs and

DOWNLOADING SOFTWARE ONLINE

Downloading software online is almost as simple as installing software from a CD-ROM or diskette. In most cases, you simply click on the appropriate link on the software's Web site to start the process. At that point, most Web browsers will then ask you where on your computer you would like to save the program. Choose a directory and then the download begins. Download times depend on the speed of your link to the online world; slower modems result in longer download times. Most useful software can be downloaded in as little as 5 or 10 minutes, but some larger applications may take up to an hour or two. Most Web browsers can usually give you a somewhat accurate estimate of the time it will take to get the software. I cannot give more step-by-step download information for the simple reason that how one does this varies greatly by computer and operating system.

Software is compressed for downloading to decrease the overall size of the downloaded file, therefore decreasing overall downloading time in the process. Software comes compressed in two main varieties for most personal computers (PC, IBM-compatible) and one variety for a Macintosh. For a PC, the program will either be an "executable" compression (the last three characters of the filename will be ".exe") or a "zipped" file (the last three characters will be ".zip"). To uncompress an executable file, all you need to do is run the program after you've downloaded and it will take you through additional installation step by step. A "zipped" file needs an "unzip" program in order to decompress the program. (A common DOS-based utility is called "pkunzip.exe" while the Windows equivalent is "WinZip." Both utilities are available from one of the general software archives listed in the section below.) Macintosh programs most often use a compression program called "StuffIt" with the "UnStuffIt" program, available at no cost.

When downloading software from the Internet, you should be aware of software viruses. Viruses are most commonly small programs that have been inserted surreptitiously into a regular piece of software. Such viruses can be playful or harmful when they run on your computer, resulting in something as simple as a clever message being displayed on your screen to your entire hard drive being erased. Care should always be taken, therefore, when downloading software. It is always safest to check all programs obtained in this manner by running a virus-checking program on the software *before* running it (but after downloading it). Such programs are available from your local computer store or for free from one of the general software catalogs listed below.

commercial versions of many pieces of software. The software developers often build into the software an expiration mechanism, so that it will expire or cease to function properly after a certain number of uses or a fixed period of time, if you do not purchase it. This gives you plenty of time to evaluate the software for your needs, and it protects the software authors from piracy and illegal use.

I've divided the following software listings into two categories. The first is mental health–related software, including psychological assessment, clinical practice, statistical, and billing software. The second category is general software. The first category I consider to be pretty comprehensive and complete as of this writing; the second category is potentially very large, so I chose a few sites, which are the largest and most popular. Some software sites offer reviews and descriptions of the programs they contain; others do not. These reviews and descriptions vary a great deal in quality and comprehensiveness. Most, however, will give you a general description of the program, its purpose, and what kind of operating systems and computers it runs on.

Because software reflects the quick changes made throughout the computer industry, any online resource which attempts to keep abreast of software programs for professionals needs to also be constantly updated. Since most Web resources available today, however, are labors of love and volunteerism for the professionals who maintain them, no site listed below for mental health-related software is comprehensive nor kept up-to-date with the latest versions of all mental health-related software available.

In addition to the sites listed bedow, Ziff-Davis has an excellent general software site which was not included in earlier printings of the book. That site may be found at `http://www.hotfiles.com/`.

Mental Health–related Software: Psychological Assessment, Clinical Practice, Statistical, and Billing Software

Title (or descriptor):   Computer Use in Social Services Network

Owner: Computer Use in Social Services Network (CUSSN)

URL (Web address):

`http://www.uta.edu/cussn/diskcopy/diskcopy.htm`

Rating: ★★

The Computer Use in Social Services Network provides a well-designed and attractive Web site to house, among other items, their "Software Connection." The Software Connection provides users with descriptions of human service freeware, shareware, and demonstration programs. The software listed on their site can be directly downloaded, or links are provided to the software's own Web site (from which it can be downloaded or purchased). Categories covered in their list include:

■ clinical and therapeutic (provides or assists in treatment or intervention)

■ welfare and child protection

■ aging

■ developmental disabilities

■ education and training

■ management

■ accounting, billing, and fund raising

■ data analysis

■ miscellaneous packages and utilities

It's a good list of programs, although it is unclear how current it is.

Title (or descriptor):   CUSSN Software Connection
Owner: Dick Shoech
URL (Web address):
      `http://www2.uta.edu/cussn/diskcopy/diskcopy.htm`
Rating: ★★

With the passing of the Computers in Mental Health (CIMH) software reviews database, finding a reliable and updated resource of computer programs of interest to clinicians and professionals is difficult. The CIMH database was especially useful because it reviewed the software it listed. Most other software listings, such as the Computer Use in Social Services Network (CUSSN) Software Connection, do not offer reviews. What the CUSSN Software Connection does offer is a fairly broad listing of software, organized into the following helpful categories: account, billing, and fund raising; aging; data analysis; developmental disabilities; education; health; management; miscellaneous; therapeutic; self-help; and welfare/child protection. While the listing isn't updated regularly, I found most of the links to be operational and with accurate but brief descriptions.

Title (or descriptor):   Kovach Computing Services (KCS)
Owner: Kovach Computing Services
URL (Web address):   `http://www.kovcomp.co.uk/`
Rating: ★★

This Web site provides customer support and information for the KCS line of inexpensive and easy-to-use statistical software. You can get the latest shareware versions through the links and order the full versions online. There are also links to other sites related to statistics and data analysis, particularly those with shareware and public domain software. The software products found on this site include: SIMSTAT for Windows, a general purpose statistical program; xlSTAT, a statistical add-in for Excel spreadsheets; MVSP, a multivariate statistical package; SIMSTAT for DOS, a general purpose statistical program for DOS; Oriana, for circular statistics; and Wa-Tor, a population dynamics simulation, among other products and services.

Title (or descriptor):   Psychology Resources
Owner: Learning and Teaching Support Network (LTSN)
URL (Web address):
        `http://www.psychology.ltsn.ac.uk/resources.html`
Rating: ★★

The potential of this Web site, which reviews not only software but also Web sites, videos, and textbooks, is that it offers the reader some insight into a particular software application before having to purchase it. This is a fairly common practice in the information technology industry, which has weekly publications reviewing new software programs in a systematic and constant manner. But in the world of psychology-related software, such up-to-date and regularly updated reviews are rare. The resource put together by LTSN suffers from its reviews' being hopelessly outdated. In the world of ever-changing software, an old review is almost worth less than no review at all because the review may contain so much misinformation as to cause an individual to make a badly informed choice. At least the site's list of programs could be used to help a researcher or clinician as a jumping off point to learning more about the software.

Title (or descriptor):	Psyc Site: Software Sites
Owner:	Department of Psychology, Nipissing University
URL (Web address):	`http://kenstange.com/psycsite/`
Rating:	★★★

Psyc Site: Software Sites is intended to point to psychology-related software available on the Internet. These links are to both shareware and commercial software. Readers may find this site helpful in locating other software archives and listings online.

Title (or descriptor):	SAS Institute
Owner:	SAS Institute, Inc.
URL (Web address):	`http://www.sas.com/`
Rating:	★★★

One of the largest statistical software developers, the SAS Institute has a thorough Web site. Although their product line is complex, they do a fairly good job in describing the individual components of the SAS software system. What they (and their competitor, SPSS) do not do is provide a simple navigational path to users who have a diverse set of needs and skillsets. A first-time user has virtually no idea which product to choose or which products offer the best solution to their needs.

Their technical support area is filled with information on how to compute various statistics with their software, as well as a comprehensive set of FAQs. Their search engine works as expected with simple keyword searches leading to a listing of results ordered in confidence level.

Title (or descriptor):	Scientific Software Catalog
Owner:	ProGAMMA
URL (Web address):	
	`http://www.progamma.nl/scien_soft/index.html`
Rating:	★★

A database of approximately 100 software programs is provided on this European site. The listings are organized either by category (such as psychological testing, biofeedback, psychological research, and multilevel analysis) or alphabetically. Reviews do mention specific software version number but are not dated, calling into question how relevant and valid they are. Prices, when available, are listed in Euros.

Title (or descriptor):	Shrinktank
Owner:	Robert Bischoff, PhD
URL (Web address):	`http://www.shrinktank.com/`
Rating:	★★

Robert Bischoff's site, which was moved from one of the earliest electronic bulletin board systems in the nation, includes an eclectic set of software under the "Downloads" option. Suffering from the same lack of information about the programs, though–with terse and sometimes cryptic descriptions–this site only gets a better rating because it has more programs to offer (over 130 at this writing). Most of these programs are shareware or freeware, and some of the files are nothing more than text files, such as an FAQ file and NIMH informational brochures taken off the Internet and other Web sites.

Title (or descriptor):	SPN Software Central
Owner:	Social Psychology Network
URL (Web address):	
	`http://www.socialpsychology.org/software.htm`
Rating:	★★★

A simple one-page list of links to software and company Web sites is divided into the following categories: data analysis; word processing, office suites, and publishing; images, animation and video; Web-related software and tutorials; miscellaneous software; and saving money on software. Psychological assessment programs are missing from this nicely organized list. It's a quick and easy way to find some of the largest, most popular software in these categories.

Title (or descriptor):	SPSS
Owner:	SPSS, Inc.

URL (Web address):   http://www.spss.com/
Rating: ★★★

Compared to the SAS Institute's home page, the SPSS home page looks cluttered and unorganized. The user is given a choice of dozens of links to choose from, with very little organization to its site index layout. The home page is also graphics-intensive and sports some graphics that look confusingly similar to banner advertisements (but are not). Like the SAS Web site, SPSS provides no clear navigational path for first-time users. A listing of all of their products on the home page gives no indication if a product matches a user's specific needs without having to walk through each product's description. This is a common corporate Web site design blunder—designing around the company's business groups or divisions, not the customer's needs or expectations.

The SPSS site is somewhat less comprehensive than the SAS site, and somewhat more difficult to navigate and use. For example, the search engine in the "SPSS AnswerNet" doesn't support a simple keyword search without first associating the search with a specific product. Their search engine interface to this database of knowledge is unnecessarily complex. Like the SAS site, SPSS supports extensive FAQs on all of their products, and provides a wealth of information and support options. Scripting resources, white papers, and real-life examples of how the software can be best utilized in different scientific disciplines.

General Software Directories

Title (or descriptor):   Jumbo
Owner: Jupitermedia Corp.
URL (Web address):   http://www.jumbo.com/
Rating: ★★

With over 300,000 shareware and freeware programs available from one location, you can't go wrong by looking at Jumbo for any application or utility you may need for your computer. Its search engine leaves a lot to be desired, however, leaving you to rely on browsing through the site's hierarchy of categories. The categories available, however, don't always lend themselves to easy browsing. For example, e-mail applications are under "Internet/Windows 95" (Macintosh users are apparently out of luck) whereas Web browsers have their own category under "Internet." Users rate software listed in the directory on a 10-point Likert scale. Short descriptions are provided for each listing, as is the date it was added, the version number, and file size.

Title (or descriptor):	Shareware.Com
Owner:	CNET Networks, Inc.
URL (Web address):	`http://www.shareware.com/`
Rating:	★★★

With over 250,000 titles to choose from, a less-annoying interface than Jumbo, fewer advertisements, more descriptions, and a more powerful search engine, Shareware.Com is a much better choice. Although offering a design that is still busy (and potentially confusing to new users), it is simple and easy to navigate. I could browse the most popular downloads arranged by operating system (or not—my choice!).

One of the nicest and most useful features of this site, beyond its comprehensive database and powerful search tools, is its download options. When you click on a file to download, it takes you to another screen that provides a list of download sites for the program. You choose the site that is geographically closest to you to ensure the fastest downloading time. Alternatively, you can use their own reliability ratings for the listed sites and choose the most reliable sites from which to download the software. It is key usability features such as this that make Shareware.Com a standout in a crowd.

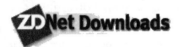

Title (or descriptor):	ZDNet Software Library
Owner:	CNET Networks, Inc.
URL (Web address):	`http://downloads-zdnet.com.com/`
Rating:	★★★★

Unlike Shareware.com and Jumbo, the ZDNet Software Library provides in-depth reviews of most of the software listed in its catalog. These reviews let you know what to expect of the freeware and shareware listed before spending the time to download it. The reviews are an invaluable addition, as it potentially can save a lot of time in evaluating new software or trying to find the right tool for your needs. In addition to the review, each software listing provides a star-review based upon the reviewer's comments, the file size, date it was added, version number, price of software (if any), and the ability to view related software titles.

The search engine was the most robust of the software directories listed here, quickly finding relevant results to search queries. Unlike the other directories, ZDNet's library doesn't attempt to be the largest. The library relies instead on choosing some of the best and most popular software titles. Its organizational scheme for categorizing software also makes the most sense. Macintosh and other computer operating system platforms, as on Shareware.com, are well supported.

CAN I USE THE INTERNET TO CHAT WITH MY COLLEAGUES ONLINE?

There are two ways you can use the Internet to chat with your colleagues, friends, or family online. One is through the use of a somewhat unreliable technology called "Internet telephony" (more commonly known as "Net-Phones"). This technology allows you to use the Internet and your computer as your telephone line and telephone, saving long distance charges. The second way to chat with people online is via "Instant Messaging" (IM) software. More about IM in a minute.

When using a NetPhone, users at either end of a connection must use the same software, and there is a fair amount of different pieces of software to choose from. Two formats are available today: audio only and audio with video. Audio only is more popular because it is less expensive, less difficult to setup, and more reliable to use, especially on slower Internet connections. Adding video with audio is a goal, but much of the technology simply isn't available or in wide enough use. If you're a technology person who has all the latest and greatest computer hardware and online connection, you may want to look into a video software package. But you must keep in mind that for it to be of real use and value to you, the person on the other end must also be able to run the same software on her machine. I won't review the available video software packages, as they are still in their infancy.

Despite all the news about NetPhones and videoconferencing software in recent years, relatively few professionals use this technology because of its complexity and lack of quality. Even as more professionals get broadband connections, I don't see this changing in the near future. The only place where such Internet telephony software is prevalent is within organizations that have telehealth or telemedicine initiatives.

The descriptions below of Internet telephone audio products were gleaned not only from my personal experiences with the software, but also from independent, third-party reviewers, such as C-Net (`http://www.cnet.com/`). All such telephony applications require that your computer have sound capabilities (e.g., a sound card in your PC) and at least a 56-Kbps modem connection to the Internet. There are no additional costs associated with the use of these applications, outside of the normal Internet connection costs you already pay. That's why these pieces of software are especially popular for people to communicate with one another across continents. Some of the products listed below may begin to approach telephone transmission quality, but most do not except under rare conditions. This is just a sample of products available; a full comparison listing of NetPhones may be found at C-Net, or at `http://www.nfe.com/owl/strouds/32phone.html`.

Using the Internet for voice communications just hasn't taken off as many people had predicted, largely because of problems of interoperability (different brands of NetPhones don't know how to communicate with one another) and poor quality. In fact, as noted below, Netscape has dropped support for a client NetPhone in its latest release of its Web browser. Instead, Netscape and other companies have seen that simple text chat is more powerful, easier to use, and more compatible with most people's computers than NetPhones have been. This movement back to basic but more widely-used communication tools online is unlikely to change in the near future.

What has taken on a life of its own are Instant Messaging (IM) applications, such as AOL's AIM and ICQ services. Instant messaging is simply being able to chat via text with others who are online the same time you are. This is typically done in a small window on your screen, through instant messaging software. The biggest drawback to these services is the same as it is for NetPhones—interoperability. It is hoped this issue will be worked out in the future, but in the meantime, ensure you are using the same software as those you want to chat with are. You may already have instant messaging software on your computer—it comes with versions of Netscape and Microsoft's Web browsers, and is a built-in feature of America OnLine.

Title (or descriptor):	AOL Instant Messenger Service (AIM)
Owner:	American OnLine
URL (Web address):	`http://www.aim.com/`

Price:	Free
System:	Any version of Windows; Mac; Linux

AOL's Instant Messenger (AIM) system is by far the industry's standard and most popular text messaging system. You do not have to use America OnLine or be a member in order to use this software. Like all instant messaging programs, AIM allows two users to "talk" to each other by typing text to one another, in real-time (both users need to be logged onto the Internet at the same time). Business users, graduate students, and teenagers use this same popular and easy-to-use technology to keep in touch with their peers. AIM is probably the easiest instant messaging software to learn, because it has a simple user interface. The single, small advertisement displayed is annoying, but doesn't really get in the way of the software's functionality.

Title (or descriptor):	CUworld
Owner:	CUworld, Inc.
URL (Web address):	`http://www.cuworld.com/`
Price:	$4.95-$14.95/month subscription
System:	Windows 98, ME, 2000, XP

The venerable free CU-SeeMe has been supplanted by commercial versions, the most well known of which resides at CUworld. (You can still find the free version to download, but its installation is much more difficult now. A business version, based on the same technology, may be found at `http://www.fvc.com/`). A lot has changed since CU-SeeMe first came on the scene a decade ago in 1994, and the technology has improved substantially. But the newer commercial versions don't support the Macintosh computer as older versions did, and the monthly subscription price quickly becomes expensive to maintain. As with any videoconferencing software, the quality of the video and audio received depend greatly on your connection speed—faster broadband connections will receive significantly higher audio and video than will dial-up connections.

Title (or descriptor):	ICQ
Owner:	ICQ, Inc.
URL (Web address):	`http://www.icq.com/`
Price:	Free
System:	Any version of Windows or Mac

Since being acquired by America OnLine, ICQ remains one of the top two most popular instant messaging applications (AOL's AIM being the other). Preferred by experienced Internet users, ICQ has many of the same features of AIM, including the ability to set up a mini chat room. ICQ relies on arbitrary numbers to identify people, which isn't as user friendly as AIM's nicknames. But the search utilities found on the ICQ Web site make it relatively easy to hunt down a person's ICQ number.

Title (or descriptor):   NetMeeting

Owner: Microsoft Corp.

URL (Web address):

`http://www.microsoft.com/windows/netmeeting/`

Price: Free

System: Any version of Windows

NetMeeting is the only product listed here that allows users to share Microsoft-based documents and spreadsheets with one another in a "whiteboard" area. Its sound quality is adequate on DSL or faster connections, but slower connection speeds (e.g., 28.8-Kbps modems) will notice especially poor quality. It is limited to users of Windows at this writing. User configuration is simple and connecting to other users is a relatively painless experience.

11

Online Therapy (E-Therapy) and Behavior

Conducting therapy online, or e-therapy, is a new experience fraught with difficulties and some lingering concerns. As of this writing, some of these concerns have been resolved through professional association guidelines, state legislatures, or other governing bodies. You would still pretty much be a virtual pioneer if you choose to pursue this modality, and, as in the real world, you may run into very real ethical and legal problems. I would caution you that this is still an emerging field, so you must be both serious and devoted to it as a viable and useful modality. You should not look at conducting online therapy just as a way to supplement your income.

While many of the particular issues—ethical and practical—of online therapy have yet to be addressed by the mental health field, one issue has been, somewhat, addressed by the field of computer-mediated communication. Some profes-

sionals argue that since a great majority of people's interactions and communication are nonverbal, any medium that is not also nonverbal will miss important body language. Others argue that since people have been utilizing the
Internet for a great deal of emotional discussion on online support groups, it
is already a benefit to many individuals online. Both viewpoints are valid.

Some forms of professional helping are readily conducted online. It is
not psychotherapy in the traditional sense, nor is it simply therapy trans-
ported to an online modality. Instead, it is apparent that it is an entirely
new modality of helping people with life problems. Just as there are benefits when people with similar disorders "talk" to one another in online support groups (sometimes referred to as "virtual support groups" in research), it follows that some type of benefit could arise from an individual
"talking" to a professional online. I leave it up to you to decide whether it
is a good idea to try out this type of online service. But if you do, keep in
mind that you are bound to the same ethical principles you hold in the
real world. This includes such requirements as stating up front the type of
service you are offering, the limits of such a service, your availability
(24 hours a day, 7 days a week? by telephone or other contact?), to what
extent your service replaces a regular therapist in the real world, and similar concerns.

Nonetheless, online therapy is still a somewhat risky venture, not only
from an ethical point of view but also from a legal one. If an individual under your care online decides to commit suicide, can the individual's family
sue you? If their heirs or family wanted to complain to a licensure board,
which board would they complain to? Would you be guilty of malpractice
for operating where you are not licensed? Who is legally empowered to
look out for and protect the patient's rights in such an instance? Can you be
brought to court for practicing in another state without a license (since your
current license probably only allows you to practice within your state of
residence)? What are the effects of offering your services to people in other
countries whose first language may not be English and who therefore may
not fully understand some of the points you are making or the terms under
which you are offering your services? What are the repercussions of offering services to someone who claims he is an adult, yet later you discover he

is a minor and you don't have parental consent to treat? As you can see, there are many legal issues to consider, some of which may seriously affect your professional reputation and ability to practice in the real world. New state laws, lawyers, and the courts will eventually decide these issues, as will the separate professional associations, who will set ethical guidelines on their profession's acceptable behaviors. Consider such ethical points carefully and check with your state licensing board, your professional liability insurance provider, as well as your national professional association to determine the current status of such laws and guidelines before offering any professional service online.

Emerging research is providing empirical support for using the Internet to conduct electronic therapy, or "e-therapy." There are now numerous case studies, of individuals and groups, benefiting from online interventions. Larger-scale studies using control groups and dozens of participants are already in the planning stages. So far, the results look promising that this new type of therapeutic modality is potentially safe and effective. It still requires a significant commitment on the part of the practitioner who wants to enter this field, because the legal and many of the ethical issues remain largely unaddressed.

I'M THINKING OF DOING SOME KIND OF THERAPY ONLINE. WHERE DO I FIND MORE INFORMATION ABOUT THE ECONOMICS, LEGALITIES, AND ETHICS OF THIS MODALITY?

Perhaps you have thought about this long and hard and have decided that online therapy is nonetheless the wave of the future. You would like to be on the cutting edge, not only of technology, but of the clinical profession as well. Where do you find information and resources about how to set up a useful online practice? There are some people who have beat you to this idea and have tried paving the way for others—you will find two such pioneers in this field below, who have been around long enough that I trust that they offer stable and reliable Web sites and, perhaps, services.

Title (or descriptor):	International Society for Mental Health Online
Owner:	International Society for Mental Health Online
URL (Web address):	http://www.ismho.org/
Rating:	★★★★

Since its inception at the end of 1997, the International Society for Mental Health Online (ISMHO) has taken the lead in establishing an open forum to discuss issues relating to the provision of online mental health services. In late 1999, it released suggested guidelines for online service providers to follow in their online practice. Growing rapidly from a small group of founding members, its membership today includes many of the pioneers in the field and representatives from national and international professional associations and companies.

Title (or descriptor):	NetPsychology
Owner:	Leonard Holmes, PhD
URL (Web address):	http://www.netpsych.com/
Rating:	★★★

This site explores the uses of the Internet to deliver mental health services and is an excellent jumping off point for professionals looking to learn more about this topic. Netpsych's owner, Leonard Holmes, is a psychologist who is careful to describe the services he offers elsewhere online ("Shareware Psychological Consultation") as *not* being therapy. He is very much aware of the legal, professional, and ethical issues involved in doing therapy online and should be considered a good resource to contact for further information. The one drawback to this site is its reliance on heavy graphics and graphical special effects, including a multitude of ads and other services, which may annoy and slow down some Web readers.

Both of these sites, along with many others, are cataloged in the "ABCs of Internet Therapy," maintained by Martha Ainsworth at `http://www.metanoia.org/imhs/`. I have also written articles regarding online counseling, which I call "e-therapy," that can be found on my Web site, Psych Central (`http://psychcentral.com/`). These kinds of resources, because they are relatively new, are not easily discovered. New resources generally don't show up in Web search engines immediately, even if a Web site author submits the information by hand to the search engines. The savvy professional, therefore, needs to know where to go to find out about new and up-and-coming resources online. I'll discuss one such option in the next section.

E-THERAPY CLINICS

E-therapy clinics offer a clinician a place and the tools to setup their online practice successfully and easily. A clinician can choose to offer e-therapy without joining such a clinic, but a clinic offers marketing, record-keeping, bookkeeping, and technology services that would be more difficult to do on your own. The downside to these clinics is that they charge for their services, sometimes including a monthly service fee no matter how much or how little business you actually do on the clinic's Web site. Keep these issues in mind when shopping around.

Title (or descriptor):	eTherapists Online
Owner:	Find-a-Therapist.com, Inc.
URL (Web address):	`http://www.etherapistsonline.com/`
Rating:	★★

A clean site design makes it straightforward and simple to schedule an online therapy session with one of the therapists from eTherapists Online. In order to join and use the service as a professional, you must pay a one-time registration fee (currently $95.00), be licensed to practice psychotherapy, and carry professional insurance. Another fee of $195.00 is required in order to set up your "virtual office," but no additional fees appear to be associated with the service.

The site suffers from a confusing array of nonintegrated services. The registration was a bit confusing, as it switched between different Web sites with different layouts, names, and menu options. Purchasing a session took me to yet a third Web site, and scheduling a session took me to a fourth Web site! This multitude of different sites, with different names and layouts, makes the process more confusing than it otherwise would be. It suggests the company is reusing different Web services it has created or contracted for for a variety of different purposes. Although, from a business perspective, this may make good financial sense, from an end-user perspective, it seems to make less sense.

The site provides a variety of modalities in which to interact with a therapist online. It is not clear from the scarce information provided on the site whether it uses encryption to protect the privacy of the therapist/client communications, or a special Web-based e-mail system when the e-mail option is chosen. Additional modalities an online client can choose from include synchronous chat and telephone callback from the therapist.

Title (or descriptor):	HelpHorizons.com
Owner:	HelpHorizons.com, Inc.
URL (Web address):	`http://www.helphorizons.com/`
Rating:	★★★

This is a site that I am an advisor for, so I cannot be completely neutral in evaluating it. It does provide its professional users a "Virtual Office" in which to set up their online practice. The tools available through this Virtual Office include secure e-mail to clients, automated record-keeping, and an integrated insurance and billing module. Professionals can also choose to use the site entirely for their regular practice only, as many of the tools are valuable for all practices.

HelpHorizons.com's e-therapy tools include secure e-mail, secure chat rooms, and secure videoconferencing, all of which is accomplished through encryption. Encryption technology protects the user's information and communications while they are sent over the Internet. The site accepts credit cards on behalf of the professional, which allows for easy payment for e-therapy by the client (as most insurance companies don't yet reimburse for these services). The professional registration process can be cumbersome, as it requires that paperwork is physically sent to the company for background verification and credentialing. Three membership levels are available, which range in cost from $20 to $40 per month, with varying levels of service.

The site is divided into two major sections—a site for consumers and a professional site. It is generally well designed with a simple, direct user interface, although its orange color may be a bit hard on some people's eyes. The consumer side of the site (to which professional members are encouraged to contribute) acts as a psychoeducational resource with hundreds of original articles. It also acts as a way of exposing consumers interested in mental health or e-therapy to the professional network of members that offer services through the site. With more than 50 professionals in its network, it is by far the largest and most established e-therapy clinic online today.

Title (or descriptor):	OnlineClinics.com
Owner:	Ron Kraus, PhD
URL (Web address):	http://www.onlineclinics.com/
Rating:	★★

Like other online clinic services, OnlineClinics.com rents virtual office space on its site and verifies the credentials of those professionals. Its online tool set appears to be smaller than that offered by HelpHorizons.com, and only a few dozen professionals are involved with the site. The site design as of this writing lacks a certain professional feel, with rotating planetary spheres and blinking navigation links throughout. Links to outside sites are contained within a frame that, while allowing easy navigation back to OnlineClinics.com's site, is considered a Web design no-no (because, for instance, it obfuscates the Web address of the site you're visiting). Outside of providing a directory to its members and links to mental health reading materials found on other Web sites, the Waiting Room section provides non-sequitor links to online games, television and radio sites, and food ordering. I found that many links in the professional directory area went nowhere, and when a professional was found, links listed on their personal page often led nowhere. A new version of the site is supposed to come online shortly, which may correct some of these problems. Varying levels of memberships are available, with fees ranging from nothing to $225 per month.

IS "INTERNET ADDICTION DISORDER" REAL? WHERE CAN I FIND ADDITIONAL INFORMATION ON THIS AND OTHER PSYCHOLOGICAL DISCUSSIONS ABOUT ONLINE BEHAVIOR?

This is an interesting and ongoing topic of debate. There is neither a single nor easy answer to this question. There exists, however, many forums that have been created to discuss this question, trade opinions and barbs among professionals, and to disseminate information. Professionals around the world are conducting research into this phenomenon, led by Kimberly Young at the University of Pittsburgh. Her Web site is listed below.

While Web sites will offer you some basic background information or point you to other online resources on the issue of the psychology of online behavior, it is in resources such as mailing lists where you will find the most lively ongoing discussions. These forums are where the majority of professionals gather to discuss this issue in-depth. A few of the most active mailing lists are listed later in this section.

Internet Addiction Web Sites

Title (or descriptor):	Center for Online Addiction
Owner:	Kimberly Young, PsyD
URL (Web address):	`http://www.netaddiction.com/`
Rating:	★★★

Kimberly Young's Center for Online Addiction has been greatly revamped and improved over time. It now offers a great deal of information about addiction and compulsive behaviors toward online use, cybersex, relationship issues, and related online issues. It also acts as a marketing tool to advertise and sell her seminars, workshops, and books related to this problem. Full-length articles about "Internet addiction" and links to other related online resources are also available.

Title (or descriptor):	Psychology of Cyberspace
Owner:	John Suler, PhD
URL (Web address):	`http://www.rider.edu/suler/psycyber/`
URL (Web address):	
	`http://www.rider.edu/suler/psycyber/resources.html`
Rating:	★★★

John Suler has put together an excellent Web site devoted to disseminating information about professionals doing research online. While discussing his own research into interactive chat and role-playing environments online, he has also collected a comprehensive listing of resources for researchers, listed in the "Other Resources" category. Here you will find a number of mailing lists and other online resources offering additional information and compelling discussion on these topics. Minimal graphics make for an easy Web site to access.

Title (or descriptor):	The Psychology of Virtual Communities
Owner:	Storm A. King
URL (Web address):	http://webpages.charter.net/stormking/
Rating:	★★★

An extensive archive of Storm King's articles, papers, and presentations about the psychology behind online communities. Although many of the resources are related to self-help support groups online, there is additional material about "Internet addiction," support for the effectiveness of online therapy, and the nature of online relationships.

Mailing List Discussions of Online Behavior

Title (or descriptor):	NetDynam—The Network Group Dynamics Mailing List
Commands to:	listserv@maelstrom.stjohns.edu
Subscribe:	subscribe netdynam Your-name
Unsubscribe:	unsubscribe netdynam
List:	netdynam@maelstrom.stjohns.edu
List owners:	Orrin Simon Onken (E-mail: simon@loris.com)

NetDynam is a small yet sometimes interesting forum which "examines and reports upon the psychological, social, philosophical and aesthetic aspects of being part of the Internet community," according to the list's welcome message. It is very much a list devoted to list dynamics, and subscribers' own reactions to other people's messages on the list. It is recommended you read the list for a while to become familiarized with the dynamics of the forum before participating in it. This is good advice to follow for any online community.

Title (or descriptor):	Philosophy and Psychology of Cyberspace
Commands to:	listserv@listserv.aol.com
Subscribe:	subscribe cybermind Your-name
Unsubscribe:	unsubscribe cybermind
List:	cybermind@listserv.aol.com
List owners:	Alan Sondheim (E-mail: sondheim@panix.com)

A strange, eclectic mailing list devoted to more philosophical issues surrounding uses of and in the online world. Just about any topic you can imagine is up for discussion and commentary. While the list's own welcome message suggests that the forum "is devoted to an examination of the new subjectivities that have emerged and might yet emerge in this [online] arena [. . .] in particular in the philosophical, psychological/psychoanalytic and social issues engendered, particularly as they concern the user and the social." If you're looking for a more philosophical discussion of the online world and its related technologies, this may be a forum to check out.

Title (or descriptor):   Psychology of the Internet: Research and Theory
URL (Web address):

    `http://groups.yahoo.com/group/psy-internet/`

Subscribe: `psy-internet-subscribe@yahoogroups.com`

Unsubscribe: `psy-internet-unsubscribe@yahoogroups.com`

List: `psy-internet@yahoogroups.com`

List owner: John M. Grohol
    (E-mail: `grohol@psychcentral.com`)

This mailing list, which I started and continue to host, tends to have a larger subscription base than other lists on this subject. This translates into more interesting and diverse discussions about the psychology of online behaviors. Unlike many other mailing lists, the complete archives of the mailing list's previous discussions are also available on the Web. This allows new subscribers to the mailing list to "catch-up" on the discussion and review what topics the list may have already addressed or covered. Sometimes mailing lists have the unfortunate tendency toward repeating the same topics. While this occurs as well on this mailing list, it seems to happen less frequently. The topic of "Internet Addiction Disorder" has been brought up multiple times on this list and some interesting theories have been discussed.

This mailing list, open to all interested professionals, discusses research and theory on the psychology of the Internet. The topics that are appropriate to this list are broadly defined, but can include such issues as how to conduct psychological research via the Internet; theory behind virtual support groups; online psychotherapy; "Internet Addiction Disorder"; the psychology of various online phenomenon, such as "flame wars," relationships, etc.

So how did I know to look at NetPsychology and other Web sites or online resources devoted to this topic? I found out about the site through a mailing list. If you're interested in this topic, you definitely should subscribe to one, or all, of them. They not only include timely and relevant discussions about research and theory online, but also announcements of new research, Web sites, and other online resources as they become available. Electronic mailing lists are still one of the best and most underrated resources available online today for finding information relevant to specific professional areas and topics.

PART III

Patient Education Resources

CHAPTER 12

General Consumer-oriented Resources on the Web

Clients and patients come to professionals for help with their disorders, and an important part of any clinical practice is the education of patients in the causes and treatments of their disorders. But clients also often want more information than the professional can readily provide. The online world has responded to this need by creating many information resources about disorders, online resources, treatment options, and much more. But because this information is often put together by people who suffer from these disorders and reflects their own individual experiences within the mental health system, it may not always be as accurate as professionals would like.

AN OVERVIEW OF PATIENT EDUCATION RESOURCES

I cannot vouch for the accuracy or integrity of all of the information that appears on all of the Web sites and online resources in this section, since they are dynamic and everchanging. I can vouch for the fact that these resources have been some of the most enduring and the most popular online, which suggests that the marketplace of online consumers and Web visitors are finding something useful to them or their problems. The usefulness may be found in the information presented; or it may be discovered in another online resource to which the site is linked; still yet, it may be that the site offers an online patient support group or information about one.

Self-help support groups have been shown to be a useful adjunctive modality in most cases, no matter what form they take. It is easy to forget that the online world offers not only the ability to "browse" but also to take part in an interactive, supportive community. The amount and degree to which self-help support resources have taken hold in the online world suggests that it is a powerful and useful modality for many, many people around the world. Online resources in the form of education and community have taken the place of self-help books for many people. They also act as an adjunct for those people already "Net savvy." Practitioners should therefore treat such resources just as they would any outside information the patient reads or learns about their disorder. Clients and laypeople can discover a wide variety of help online through the resources below. They are listed here to allow you to direct your clients and patients, who may have online access, to useful and popular Web sites on their disorder.

So why do people turn to online self-help support resources in the first place? Individuals who live in remote or rural areas, for instance, may not have access to good-quality or affordable mental health care. There may also simply not be enough people in their local community to create a real-world support group. Getting online offers such individuals the opportunity to ask questions of professionals and participate in online support groups. Others may have difficulty in social relationships in the real world and find that starting out such friendships online may help them progress in their own real-life relationships. It is also the reward of discovering that one is not alone with one's thoughts and feelings, and the feeling of community that the online world can support and nurture in these individuals. This process of seeking community and like-minded individuals with which to discuss specific topics is mirrored in the reasons professionals, too, get online. Last, many people still feel the stigma attached to mental illness. Online, there is much less stigmatization of such problems.

MAKING THE MOST OF OUTSIDE MATERIALS

Patients have always brought outside materials to therapy sessions to share them with the practitioner. These range from a newspaper clipping about their disorder, to a book they have read and found valuable, to brochures or pamphlets published on their problem. Clinicians should take an objective and unbiased position on such materials, helping the patient understand the information in the context of the patient's presentation of the disorder and what the scientific research currently tells us about the disorder. Such a discussion is often beneficial on a number of different levels: It allows the patient to become a better-educated consumer of mental health problems and therapies; and such a discussion can open up avenues of exploration within therapy, or correct common misconceptions about what is currently known about the causes and treatment of mental disorders.

As it becomes more common for people to get online, some of your patients will want to share with you material they have come across in their online travels. This may include offerings on new treatments for their disorder, but unique additions as well. For instance, it may not be uncommon to have a patient come into a therapy session with a transcript of an online interactive chat they had with another person or professional. The patient may want to share what was learned in this interaction, or ask questions that the interaction raised in the patient's mind. A clinician can effectively incorporate this type of material into their therapy with the client by examining the meaning of the interaction. There is an endless array of possibilities such material may help uncover in therapy. The material, therefore, should be treated with all the seriousness and objectivity that any written material brought into therapy would be. Some skepticism, however, may not be inappropriate, given the anonymity of online interactions, especially if the patient is not familiar with or does not know the other online person very well. Examining the quality of the interaction, the type of content discussed, and the manner in which the people in the interaction related to one another will help you make the most of the material presented.

Naturally such material should never become the sole focus of therapy. Clinicians should be wary of clients focusing extensively or exclusively on their online interactions, especially if doing so is at the expense of real-world interactions with family members, coworkers, and friends. As with the discussion of any material brought into therapy to be shared with the practitioner, it should be done in a manner that is conducive to elaborating existing therapeutic issues and goals. It should not be used as an excuse by the patient—or the therapist—to keep from focusing on the issues of relevance within therapy.

Education, community, togetherness, and acceptance. Excellent reasons that your patients may want to utilize the online world to their advantage and take an active role in their treatment. This section will help you help your clients, by describing and reviewing resources likely to be most relevant to your clients' problems. As with all sections in this book, look for updates to the information listed here (such as new Web sites or other online resources which I believe may be important to visit) at the book's Web site (`http://www.insidemh.com/`).

There are thousands of consumer-oriented Web sites that disseminate information about mental disorders online. Many of these include not only general information about the disorder itself (such as common symptoms), but may host a frequently asked questions (FAQ) file about the disorder as well. Poems, personal stories of coping with the disorder in their lives, Web-based discussion forums, real-world resources, and contact information and links to other online resources round out many of these sites.

Because of the multitude of these resources online, I felt it would be nearly impossible to list them all here and unfair to select which disorders should be represented. Instead, I will list some of the larger, more general mental health sites on the Web. Since the Web is very easy to get around on, you can point a patient to one of these general resources, and he will be able to quickly find more specific information and additional links to his disorder. Some of the following are guides that act as indices to other online resources. Other listings below are sites that contain information about disorders themselves. The type of site (listed in alphabetical order below) is listed in the description.

 American Psychiatric Association

Title (or descriptor):	American Psychiatric Association
Owner:	American Psychiatric Association
URL (Web address):	`http://www.psych.org/`
Rating:	★★★★
Type:	Informational site

A great deal of information about mental disorders may be found directly on this site, especially in their "Let's Talk Facts" brochure series. These brochures address most major mental disorders in depth, in an easy-to-read style and without a lot of "psychobabble." The information presented is relatively balanced and shouldn't offend most mental health professionals in the conclusions drawn or recommendations of treatment modalities. The site is attractive and easy to navigate.

Title (or descriptor):	APA HelpCenter
Owner:	American Psychological Association
URL (Web address):	`http://helping.apa.org/`
Rating:	★★★
Type:	Informational site

The consumer information provided on the HelpCenter is neither as comprehensive nor as helpful as that found on the American Psychiatric Association's Web site. Divided into three main categories, "Psychology at Work," "Mind/Body Connection," and "Family and Relationships," few of the articles listed discuss specific mental disorders or concerns. Subcategories, such as "How to Find Help for Life's Problems" and "Get the Facts," are nothing more than thinly veiled advertisements for the benefits of psychotherapy. Filled with a healthy dose of truisms, the site's design is mediocre. For example, it took four clicks from the home page to find a relevant article on relationships; their idea of a guestbook is really nothing more than a feedback form.

Title (or descriptor):	At Health
Owner:	At Health, Inc.
URL (Web address):	`http://www.athealth.com/`
Rating:	★★★
Type:	Informational site

Just as its clinician's site has gradually emerged as a leading resource over the past few years, At Health's consumer site has also taken on a life of its own. Its content covers all the major (and many minor) mental health issues and disorders, written in accessible language for the average consumer. In addition to a description of the problem, treatment and self-help solutions are also provided, making At Health's content a well-rounded resource for clients. Featured articles on the site provide additional original information, highlighting a specific area of concern every month. The Resource Center displays a listing of real-world community resources relating to specific concerns, as well as some online resources. A bookstore, drug database, and a self-help products store round out the major offerings available on this site. Its clean interface, largely devoid of advertising, is a refreshing change in an increasingly cluttered online world, but the site could benefit from the addition of an internal search engine.

Title (or descriptor):	Go Ask Alice
Owner:	Healthwise, Columbia University
URL (Web address):	http://www.goaskalice.columbia.edu/
Rating:	★★★★
Type:	Informational site

A service of the Columbia University Healthwise program, this site is mainly oriented toward students. However, the sensible information on sexuality, sexual health, general health, alcohol and other drugs, fitness and nutrition, emotional well-being, and relationships is general enough that nearly anybody can benefit from reading through this attractive and content-rich site.

Title (or descriptor):	Mental Health Matters
Owner:	Get Mental Help, Inc.
URL (Web address):	http://www.mental-health-matters.com/
Rating:	★★
Type:	Guide and informational site

Apparently still under development, this site offers the usual array of symptom lists, disorder information, treatment types, and related Internet resources. Most articles are sourced on the site, but few carry dates and many seem to be simply reprints from other sites. Advertising overwhelms the site's content; I counted at least seven separate advertisements on most pages. A "Related articles" table next to most articles on the site wasn't very good at determining relevant content.

Title (or descriptor):	Mental Help Net
Owner:	CenterSite, LLC
URL (Web address):	`http://mentalhelp.net/`
Rating:	★★★
Type:	Guide & Informational site

This mental health subject guide offers thousands of links to online resources, which may help patients to better understand and gain support in coping with their disorder. Comprehensive and large in nature, it reviews many of the sites listed within its database to help readers discover whether a resource is worth looking at. Mental Help Net houses the American Self-Help Clearinghouse's *Self-Help Sourcebook Online* (`http://mentalhelp.net/selfhelp`), a massive database of self-help organizations throughout the world. *Psychological Self-Help*, a 1,000-page self-help book, is available here as well (`http://mentalhelp.net/psyhelp/`). This book offers hundreds of insights and tips for consumers on how to deal with many common mental disorders and, like everything else on Mental Help Net, is completely searchable. Its ability to keep up to date in the past few years has lagged far behind the Internet's growth. With its limited resources, it now contains many outdated resources and links that lead to nowhere.

Title (or descriptor):	National Alliance for the Mentally Ill
Owner:	National Alliance for the Mentally Ill (NAMI)
URL (Web address):	`http://www.nami.org/`
Rating:	★★★
Type:	Informational site

The National Alliance for the Mentally Ill (NAMI) has greatly broadened its online efforts in recent years, branching out from a simple informational and advocacy Web site. In addition to its usual offering of informational pamphlets, it now offers consumers online communities for schizophrenia, depression, bipolar disorder, anxiety disorders, obsessive-compulsive disorder, and other mental illnesses. These communities provide online discussion forums, updated news, book reviews, spotlight articles, and fact sheets. Keeping in mind NAMI's historic bias of viewing these disorders as primarily biologically based, their Web site is a growing resource worthy of consideration.

Title (or descriptor):   National Institute of Mental Health

Owner: National Institute of Mental Health (NIMH)

URL (Web address):   `http://www.nimh.nih.gov/`

Rating: ★★★

Type: Informational site

The National Institute of Mental Health's Web site has drastically improved over the past year. The always-useful content is now provided in a more readable and consumer-friendly (but still plain) format. An overly complex search engine allows searching for topics on its and the National Institutes of Health Web sites. Aspects of NIMH's content are becoming outdated, sorely needing updates to reflect the latest knowledge and research in mental disorders.

Title (or descriptor):   National Mental Health Association

Owner: National Mental Health Association

URL (Web address):   `http://www.nmha.org/`

Rating: ★★★

Type: Informational site

With topics covered in advocacy, outreach, prevention, and general information about mental disorders and mental health issues, this site will improve as it places more of its balanced fact sheets online.

Title (or descriptor):   Psych Central

Owner: John M. Grohol, PsyD

URL (Web address):   `http://psychcentral.com/`

Rating: ★★★

Type: Guide and informational site

A resource guide to thousands of mental health and psychology resources online, Psych Central also offers an extensive article library on mental health and relationship concerns. Symptom lists, interactive online quizzes, an active self-help support community, a Web log (or "blog"), and daily-updated news feeds from around the Web round out my personal offering to the world of online mental health and psychology.

Title (or descriptor):   Psych Web

Owner: Russ Dewey

URL (Web address):   http://www.psychwww.com/

Rating: ★★

Type: Guide

A very good subject guide not only for those interested in psychology, but for anyone who is looking for additional information on psychological and mental health topics. The "Self-Help Resources on the Web" category contains a large listing of online resources for those looking for specific disorder information. This resource is apparently updated very irregularly.

Title (or descriptor):   Psychology Information Online

Owner: Donald J. Franklin, PhD

URL (Web address):   http://www.psychologyinfo.com/

Rating: ★★★

The title of this resource is deceptive, because Psychology Information Online contains information on a great deal more than just psychology. Much of the information is written by psychologist Donald Franklin, who covers topics such as mental health disorders, types of treatments, comparing types of doctors, a forensic psychology section, a bookstore, and a solid FAQ (Frequently Asked Questions) file about psychologists. Information is supplemented with links to other reliable sites, such as the National Institute of Mental Health. This site appears to be constantly growing and offers information relevant not only to consumers, but also professionals.

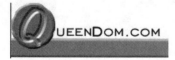

Title (or descriptor):   Queendom.com

Owner: Plumeus, Inc.

URL (Web address):   http://www.queendom.com/

Rating: ★★★★

Queendom.com is an established mental health Web site that, despite it's odd name, has a new lease on life. It has always been known as a place to go for online quizzes (and, in fact, serves as the impetus for the more professionally oriented site, PsychTests.com, reviewed in Chapter 3). With its most recent redesign, the site offers an even broader mix of interactive tests and quizzes (nearly 400) of both the "just-for-fun" variety as well as serious psychometric instruments. The advice and knowledge sections have been organized and expanded, however, now offering hundreds of articles on topics of mental health, relationships, and women's health. What's refreshing about Queendom.com is its focus not so much on a problem-solution approach toward mental health, but a broader attitude celebrating health and healthy living more so than most mental health sites.

A thriving discussion forum community is also in evidence here, using software that is one of the most user-friendly available from any of the larger mental health Web sites. Topics covered within the community reflect the larger topic area covered by the site, such as emotional health, women's health, relationships, and general health. Some of the boards have thousands of messages in them, contributed by hundreds of community members. This is a site that is both fun and informative—a combination rarely achieved.

13

Online Consumer Discussion and Support Groups

There is a wealth of discussion and support groups online for consumers. In fact, the original reason I became excited about mental health online was coming across just such a group, alt.support.depression (an Internet newsgroup) during the summer of 1991. I stumbled across this peer-run support group quite by accident, however. I was frustrated by my experience in trying to locate similar types of groups on the Internet at the time, so I began compiling and maintaining a list of mental health and psychology discussion groups online. And the rest, as they say, is history.

Discussion and support on the Internet is carried out in three central locations: on mental health Web sites, on mailing lists, and on newsgroups. This chapter will briefly describe how to go about finding some of the resources available for each modality, and provide examples of each modality. The most popular modality of support online in the early 1990s was newsgroups (before the Web), because they were a long-established technology used for online interactive discussion. Their use has declined in recent years, as more people have turned to the less-congested and higher-quality content of support groups found on Web sites and on mailing lists. Some of the strongest thriving online communities can be found in these places, and they are positive resources to refer clients to as an adjunctive support to treatment.

Like their real-world counterparts, most online consumer support groups are peer-led, and professionals are usually discouraged from participating in the group (unless they are there as a fellow consumer to address the same types of issues). It's not that professionals' views aren't valuable, just that they aren't appropriate for a peer-led support group! Consumers use these groups as a way of exchanging support and information about their disorder. Sometimes they use them as a means of venting off steam about their treatment providers, or looking for a source of a second opinion about their issues. Most groups also have a large social component, and in the more cohesive, close-knit groups, many members become close friends. One thing to remember about these groups is that they offer the potential for community and social support for an individual, but they in no way guarantee it. Just like in the real-world, the benefits obtained through an online group are largely dependent upon what the person contributes to it.

COMMUNITY MENTAL HEALTH WEB SITES

Similar to the resources listed in Chapter 12, there are a few larger mental health Web sites that offer an online community. Each of these sites has its strengths and weaknesses; only by visiting one will an individual be able to decide if the fit is right for him or her. Most of these sites' forums are monitored by volunteer or professional staff, but usually not 24 hours a day. The quality of the communities themselves, putting aside the technologies that are used to support them, is largely dependent upon the people who decide to frequent the groups. While there are usually "regulars" in any group, community Web sites seem to go through their share of regular members more often than other group modalities. This turnover may be related to the transient, click-as-you-go nature of Web surfing behavior, but whatever the reason, it usually makes for less group cohesion over the long term.

Title (or descriptor):	Dr. Grohol's Forums
Owner:	PsychCentral.com
URL (Web address):	`http://forums.grohol.com/`
Rating:	★★★

Please see the review of this active online self-help support community that I maintain in the previous section. With over 3,000 members and a dozen forums on mental health topics, it is a safe online community where members help one another with advice and support.

Title (or descriptor):	HealingWell.com Community
Owner:	HealingWell.com
URL (Web address):	`http://community.healingwell.com/community/`
Rating:	★★★

HealingWell.com is a vibrant, active online self-help support community that features forums for both health and mental health issues. Although the site offers over two dozen forums, only about a half dozen are mental health related. The forum software provides community members with a wealth of features that most people have come to expect in an online community (such as private messaging and a community events calendar). The 4,000+ membership appears to be largely supportive of one another in the forums, which are active without being overwhelming in the amount of traffic.

Title (or descriptor):	HealthyPlace
Owner:	HealthyPlace.com, Inc.
URL (Web address):	`http://www.healthyplace.com/`
Rating:	★★★

HealthyPlace is a site that originated by bringing together a set of consumer-run Web sites on various mental health topics under one umbrella. By combining individual efforts into one larger group effort, they cleverly leveraged the increased traffic levels to begin a thriving mental health community. The site's strength lies in its chat rooms, well visited with dozens of people in them throughout the day and night. The chat rooms host support groups scheduled throughout the week, on topics such as eating disorders and depression support. I liked the site so much, I host my weekly mental health Q&A chat at it! Its discussion forums are its weakest point, with a user interface that is poorly designed and requiring a great many clicks to read an entire thread of messages.

Title (or descriptor):	MentalEarth Community
Owner:	Warren Selekman, PhD
URL (Web address):	`http://www.mentalearth.com/`
Rating:	★★★

When Mental Help Net shut down its community in 2002, a lot of long-time supporters of the message boards online felt the effects. Warren Selekman, who was overseeing the Mental Help Net community, decided to take matters into his own hands and opened up his own independent mental health support groups at MentalEarth Community. This growing community site has over 800 members and over three dozen different forums ranging from the serious and supportive, to the lighter and more social.

MAILING LISTS

There are hundreds of support and discussion mailing list groups devoted to health and mental health issues, far too many to list in a book such as this. Medical disease support—getting emotional support from others who have experienced the same disease, such as cancer—is a popular category in this area. But mental health issues, too, take up a large number of groups.

When searching for a support mailing list at a site like Yahoo! Groups, keep in mind that a search on a single keyword such as "depression" will return nearly 1,000 results and not be of much use. Instead, narrow your search just as you would in a regular search engine, by using phrases (enclosed in quotation marks) or additional keywords. For instance, you might try two keywords together, like "depression support" or "childhood depression" to narrow your search.

There are two other key things to look for when choosing a support mailing list. Look for groups with larger memberships. This is contrary to real-world therapy or support groups. An online support group with only 20 members isn't likely to be of much value compared to one with 200 members. Why? Because many people in these groups do not contribute much to the group. They are referred to as "lurkers," indicating their tendency to stay in the background and just read other people's contributions. Online groups typically have a large percentage of lurkers, often up to 90% of the group's membership. A larger group makes it more likely the group will have a solid stream of conversation and various personalities to keep it cohesive and useful. (This is true up to a point! Anything much over 300 members is probably too much to handle for most people.) The second item to look for in an online group is when the last post was made to the group. A group that hasn't had any activity for a few months isn't likely to be of much value to someone looking for support or help.

Mailing lists, unlike newsgroups or many Web sites, come and go more often. To find a support group online, visit one of the large, general mailing list providers such as Yahoo! Groups (`http://groups.yahoo.com/`) or Topica (`http://www.topica.com/`) and type in appropriate keywords to find a relevant group. A smaller sampling of only mental health and disease support groups can also be found on my Web site, Psych Central (`http://www.psychcentral.com/`). You can also use your favorite search engine to find an online support group, such as Google (`http://www.google.com/`). Just form a specific query as described earlier, such as "depression support mailing list" or "depression support subscribe" or "depression online support group." Queries such as these provide quick but relevant results relating to online support groups related to depression.

NEWSGROUPS

Newsgroups can be an excellent forum for patients to engage in lively discussions and gain support and information. They are listed in alphabetical order in the table beginning on the next page. For an up-to-date listing, please consult Psych Central:

`http://psychcentral.com/`

or on the book's Web site,

`http://www.insidemh.com/`

TABLE 13.1   Patient-oriented Newsgroups

Description	Newsgroup Name	Moder-ated?
Abortion: Support for those who have had or are going to have an abortion, and their partners	alt.support.abortion	No
Abuse offenders/perpetrators, recovery for	alt.abuse.offender.recovery	No
Abuse, alternative models of dealing with	alt.abuse.transcendence	No
Abuse, moderated version of alt.sexual.abuse.recovery	alt.sexual.abuse.recovery.moderated	Yes
Abuse, recovering from all types of	alt.abuse.recovery	No
Adoptees	soc.adoption.adoptees	No
Adoption information & parenting issues	alt.adoption.agency	No
Adoption issues, general	alt.adoption	No
AIDS & HIV, general discussion of	misc.health.aids	No
AIDS & HIV, medical discussion of	sci.med.aids	Yes
AIDS, partners of people with	alt.support.aids.partners	No
All other support topics & questions	alt.support	No
Allergies, causes and treatment of	alt.med.allergy	No
Allergies, Individuals with food	alt.support.food-allergies	No
Angst	alt.angst	No
Anxiety and panic disorders	alt.support.anxiety-panic	No
Anxiety and panic disorders, cognitive approaches to	alt.recovery.panic-anxiety.self-help	No
Attention-deficit disorders	alt.support.attn-deficit	No
Breastfeeding	alt.support.breastfeeding	No
Breast implants, people with or considering	alt.support.breast-implant	No
Cancer	alt.support.cancer	No
Cancer, medical discussion of	sci.med.diseases.cancer	No
Cerebral palsy	alt.support.cerebral-palsy	No
Childless by choice	alt.support.childfree	No
Children's health issues	misc.kids.health	No

TABLE 13.1 (continued)

Description	Newsgroup Name	Moderated?
Children's issues, general	`misc.kids`	No
Chronic Fatigue Syndrome (CFS)	`alt.med.cfs`	Yes
Chronic pain	`alt.support.chronic-pain`	No
Codependency	`alt.recovery.codependency`	No
Crisis situations	`soc.support.depression.crisis`	No
Crohn's/ulcerative colitis/irritable bowel	`alt.support.crohns-colitis`	No
Cults: Former cult members & family & friends	`alt.support.ex-cult`	No
Dentistry, medical discussion of	`sci.med.dentistry`	No
Depressed people, family & friends coping with	`soc.support.depression.family`	No
Depression & mood disorders	`alt.support.depression`	No
Depression & mood disorders	`soc.support.depression.misc`	No
Depression, treatment of	`soc.support.depression.treatment`	No
Developmental delay	`alt.support.dev-delays`	No
Diabetes, hypoglycemia (hypoglycaemia)	`misc.health.diabetes`	No
Diabetes, parents & family of children with	`alt.support.diabetes.kids`	No
Dieting through medication	`alt.support.diet.rx`	No
Dieting with Weight Watchers	`alt.support.diet.weight-watcher`	No
Dieting/losing weight/nutrition	`alt.support.diet`	No
Disabled persons discussing sexuality	`alt.support.disabled.sexuality`	No
Disabled persons who are also artists	`alt.support.disabled.artists`	No
Dissociative disorders (e.g., multiple personality disorder)	`alt.support.dissociation`	No
Divorce/marital breakups	`alt.support.divorce`	No
Dwarfism	`alt.support.dwarfism`	Yes
Eating disorders (anorexia, bulimia, etc.)	`alt.support.eating-disord`	No
Effects of second-hand smoke	`alt.support.non-smokers`	No
Endometriosis	`alt.support.endometriosis`	No
Epilepsy	`alt.support.epilepsy`	No

TABLE 13.1   (continued)

Description	Newsgroup Name	Moder-ated?
Fat people, self-acceptance with no diet talk	`soc.support.fat-acceptance`	No
Fat-acceptance with no dieting talk	`alt.support.big-folks`	No
Fibromyalgia fibrosis	`alt.med.fibromyalgia`	No
Food addiction and compulsive eating	`alt.recovery.compulsive-eat`	No
Foster parents	`alt.support.foster-parents`	No
Gay youths helping each other	`soc.support.youth.gay-lesbian-bi`	Yes
Grief and loss	`alt.support.grief`	No
Headache and migraine ailments	`alt.support.headaches.migraine`	No
Hearing loss and the hearing-impaired	`alt.support.hearing-loss`	No
Height, people far from average	`alt.sigma2.height`	No
Herpes	`alt.support.herpes`	No
Hypnosis	`alt.hypnosis`	No
Infertility, causes & treatment of	`alt.infertility`	No
Learning disabilities (e.g., dyslexia)	`alt.support.learning-disab`	No
Loneliness	`alt.support.loneliness`	No
Loneliness	`soc.support.loneliness`	Yes
Looking after & taking care of another	`alt.support.disabled.caregivers`	No
Manic depression & bipolar disorder	`soc.support.depression.manic`	No
Manic depression & bipolar disorder	`alt.support.depression.manic`	No
Marfan syndrome	`alt.support.marfan`	No
Marriage	`alt.support.marriage`	No
Medicine & related products & regulations	`sci.med`	No
Menopause	`alt.support.menopause`	No
Mental health issues in society	`alt.society.mental-health`	No
Miscarriages and coping with loss in pregnancy	`soc.support.pregnancy.loss`	No
Multiple sclerosis	`alt.support.ms-recovery`	No
Multiple sclerosis	`alt.support.mult-sclerosis`	No
Muscular dystrophy	`alt.support.musc-dystrophy`	No

TABLE 13.1   (continued)

Description	Newsgroup Name	Moder-ated?
Neurological disorders	`alt.support.disorders.neurological`	No
Nicotine help	`alt.recovery.nicotine`	No
Nutrition & diet, medical discussion	`sci.med.nutrition`	No
Obesity	`alt.support.obesity`	Yes
Obsessive–compulsive disorder (OCD)	`alt.support.ocd`	No
Oppositional defiant disorder	`alt.support.opp-defiant`	No
Parenting: raising twins and other multiples	`alt.parenting.twins-triplets`	No
Parenting and adoption issues	`soc.adoption.parenting`	No
Parenting help & solutions	`alt.parenting.solutions`	No
Parenting, help being a step-parent	`alt.support.step-parents`	No
Parenting, single parenting solutions & support	`alt.support.single-parents`	No
Parenting, spanking	`alt.parenting.spanking`	No
Parenting, support and information for single fathers	`alt.dads-rights`	Yes
Personality disorders	`alt.support.personality`	No
Pet loss	`alt.support.grief.pet-loss`	No
Post polio syndrome	`alt.support.post-polio`	No
Pregnancy & childbirth issues	`misc.kids.pregnancy`	No
Procrastination help	`alt.recovery.procrastinate`	No
Prostate cancer	`alt.support.cancer.prostate`	No
Prostatitis	`alt.support.prostate.prostatitis`	No
Psychological problems, general help with	`alt.psychology.help`	No
Recovering adults from dysfunctional families	`alt.recovery.adult-children`	No
Recovering from gambling addictions	`alt.recovery.addiction.gambling`	No
Recovering from sexual abuse	`alt.sexual.abuse.recovery`	No
Recovering from sexual abuse discussion	`alt.sexual.abuse.recovery.d`	No
Recovering from sexual addictions	`alt.recovery.addiction.sexual`	No
Recovering from the effects of religion	`alt.recovery.religion`	No

TABLE 13.1   (continued)

Description	Newsgroup Name	Moder-ated?
Recovery from Catholic upbringing	`alt.recovery.catholicism`	No
Recovery issues, general	`alt.recovery`	No
Recovery through Alcoholics Anonymous	`alt.recovery.aa`	No
Recovery through Narcotics Anonymous	`alt.recovery.na`	No
Repetitive strain injuries	`misc.health.injuries.rsi.misc`	No
Repetitive strain injuries	`misc.health.injuries.rsi.moderated`	Yes
Schizophrenia support and information	`alt.support.schizophrenia`	No
Seasonal affective disorder	`soc.support.depression.seasonal`	No
Seasonal affective disorder (SAD)	`alt.support.depression.seasonal`	No
Self-improvement tips & techniques	`alt.self-improve`	No
Sex reassignment surgery or procedures, people going through	`alt.support.sexreassign`	No
Sexual abuse survivors, partners of	`alt.support.abuse-partners`	No
Short people, issues of interest to	`alt.support.short`	No
Shyness	`alt.support.shyness`	No
Sleep disorders & problems sleeping	`alt.support.sleep-disorder`	No
Smoking, stopping or quitting	`alt.support.stop-smoking`	No
Smoking like above, but moderated	`alt.support.non-smokers.moderated`	Yes
Spina bifida	`alt.support.spina-bifida`	No
Stuttering & other speaking difficulties	`alt.support.stuttering`	No
Suicide discussion	`alt.suicide.holiday`	No
Survivors of Prozac & other SSRIs	`alt.support.survivors.prozac`	No
Tall people, issues of interest to	`alt.support.tall`	No
Tinnitus/ringing ears/other head noises	`alt.support.tinnitus`	No
Tourette's syndrome	`alt.support.tourette`	No
Transgendered & intersexed persons	`soc.support.transgendered`	No
Trauma and PTSD (posttraumatic stress disorder)	`alt.support.trauma-ptsd`	No

PART **IV**

Appendices

APPENDIX A
Glossary of Terms

This is a glossary of technical terms discussed throughout this book. It has been compiled from a wide variety of sources and reflects my current knowledge.

blog *See* **Web log.**

bookmark An option within your Web **browser** that allows you to save the name and address of a Web site for future reference and easy access. Also referred to as "favorites" or "favorite places."

Boolean See **operator.**

bps, bits per second A measurement of data transmission speed particularly over a **modem.** Most popular modems transmit at either 14.4 Kbps (14,400 bps) or 28.8 Kbps (28,800 bps). Newer modems are capable of 33.6 Kbps and 56 Kbps. Some special modems may go up to 128 Kbps (over **ISDN** telephone lines).

browser Also known as a "Web browser." Any program used to access and search the World Wide Web. For instance, Netscape Navigator or Communicator, Microsoft Explorer, Mosaic, Lynx, etc.

cable modem A piece of computer hardware which gives a user high-speed access to the Internet, through your existing T.V. cable connection.

closed Used to refer to a type of mailing list. A closed mailing list only allows members of the mailing list to send messages to it. *See also* **open** and **moderated.**

COM port Serial port for connecting a cable to an IBM PC-compatible computer, usually, but not always used for data communications. They are referred to by the operating system as COM1, COM2, COM3, etc.

conference A group of public messages on a system, usually focused on a particular topic and sometimes moderated by a conference host or moderator who guides the discussion. Also called "forums," "folders," "message boards," "boards," or "SIGs" (for Special Interest Groups"). Very similar to the newsgroups on the Internet, conference is another term for public, topical, threaded discussion areas.

crawlers   The software used to index the World Wide Web. Also called "robots" and "spiders."

domain   An organization's name on the Internet. The last two parts of an e-mail address or an URL are referred to as a "domain." For example, "`aol.com`" refers to America OnLine, "`harvard.edu`" refers to Harvard University, and "`cape.org`" refers to the Cape Cod Institute.

download   Transfering files or software from another computer to your computer.

DSL, **digital subscriber line**   A service that provides high-speed Internet access through a person's regular telephone line. Is comparable and the direct competitor to a **cable modem** in terms of offering high-speed Internet access.

e-mail   Electronic mail–messages can be sent anywhere in the world via the Internet at the cost of a local phone call. E-mail addresses generally consist of a part of your name (or your account name), the "at" sign (@), followed by your domain name. For example, `webmaster@cmhc.com` is a valid e-mail address. For most e-mail addresses, it does not matter if the letters are upper- or lowercase (that is, e-mail addresses are not case-sensitive).

encryption   A secure method of encoding data, most often through a Web page or e-mail. This encoded data can only be decoded by the person or computer system authorized to access it. Used on the Web to protect financial information.

e-therapy   Another term for online counseling or online therapy. A new modality of providing helping services to people online through e-mail, forums, audio/video, or chat rooms.

FAQ   Frequently Asked Questions–A file established for many public discussion groups containing common questions new users often ask and answers to those questions.

favorite places   *See* **bookmark**.

flame   An angry, often abusive and denigrating message sent in response to another message in a public discussion forum online. Sending a flame, or "flaming" another, is frowned on and should be avoided.

form   A form is a Web page with areas you fill out (called "fields") with requested information. Forms are used to submit search queries, feedback, and requests for additional information on many Web sites.

forums   *See* **conference.**

frame   Also known as "framed." A framed Web site is one that divides your Web browser's screen into smaller areas. Each area is then filled in with different information, often in an attempt to help you navigate the Web site or to display advertising.

ftp, file transfer protocol   The standard method for transfering files over the Internet or the software program that implements this method. Using an ftp software program, you can connect to another computer online and transfer files to your local desktop computer using a GET command. Many sites allow "anonymous" ftp. At the login prompt, enter "anonymous" as the login name (without the quotes), and at the password prompt enter your e-mail address as the password. You will have access to a limited number of public directories from which you can retrieve files.

GIF, graphical interface format   A standard graphics or image file widely used on the Web. Typically works best when the graphic or image is not a photograph. *See also* **JPEG.**

gopher   The precursor to the World Wide Web. A storage-and-retrieval protocol for text and software files on the Internet. It makes finding files and useful information easier than with ftp, but harder than through the Web.

guide   A general or specialized index of online resources (most often Web sites) compiled by human editors. Less comprehensive than many search engines, but often more to the point. Also called a "search" or "subject guide."

hard drive   Your computer's internal storage device in which you save data, files, and programs.

hit   A single access of a Web page, recorded each time a Web browser displays a page. Counting the number of hits a particular Web page receives is a popularly displayed number on many people's home pages. Webmasters use hits to determine which pages are most popular and therefore should receive the most attention.

home page or **homepage**   The top-level hypertext document in a hierarchical collection of linked HTML documents. The home page is often the document implied in a WWW site's URL. For instance, `http://www.behavior.net/` actually pulls up that site's home page document, `http://www.behavior.net/index.html`.

HTML, Hypertext Markup Language   The publishing standard used to create WWW pages. It defines what happens when one clicks on a **hypertext link** embedded in the page. HTML is a publishing standard, not a programming language, hence its ease of use. HTML documents go to make up the core of a Web site, and usually end with a `.html` or `.htm` suffix.

HTTP, Hypertext Transfer Protocol   The standard by which the World Wide Web operates.

hypertext link   Also known as a "link," it is often displayed as highlighted and underlined text on a Web page; graphics can also be links, however. By choosing a hypertext link (by clicking on it with your mouse), you are instructing the computer to go to and display a specific Web document. This allows individuals to move within a Web site, or across Web sites residing on different computers, with ease. A "bad" link is one that does not work properly. When a bad link is encountered, you will receive an error message instead of the Web page you were trying to visit. Links become bad most often because a Web page has moved (and has left no forwarding address) or because the page was simply removed from the Web.

Internet   The largest global network of business and personal computers connected through regular and high-speed telephone lines. Requires specific types of software to access it, such as a Web browser.

IP, Internet Protocol   An alternative method for accessing Web sites, based on the Web site's technical address. This takes the form of a four-part number, such as 207.87.223.39.

ISDN, Integrated Services Digital Network   An all-digital telephone system slowly gaining more use and acceptance throughout the United States, ISDN allows individuals to use higher speed modems than standard telephone lines. Requires specialized installation and equipment at the present time.

Java, Javascript   These are two separate but related, largely Web-based programming languages. They allow for increased functionality of and enhancements to a Web site. If your browser is not capable of using these languages, the enhancements or features found in the Web site will most often simply not be displayed. Netscape and Microsoft support both types of languages.

JPEG, Joint Photographic Experts Group   A standard for compressing digital photographic images. *See also* **GIF**.

Kb, Kilobyte   1,024 bytes; often generically applied to 1,000 bytes as well.

link   *See* **hypertext link**.

mailing list A public, topical discussion group that is conducted exclusively through e-mail. Once a user subscribes to a mailing list, any messages she subsequently sends to the list are copied and re-distributed to every other user on the mailing list. A common way to carry on topic-specific discussions online; the other is via **newsgroups**. Mailing lists are also sometimes known as "listservs" or "majordomos," named after the types of software used to maintain them.

Mb, Megabyte Technically 1,024 kilobytes or 1,048,576 bytes, but often applied to the more rounded term of 1 million bytes as well.

mirror A Web site that duplicates another Web site at a different physical location. Often done to help speed access to that resource because it resides on another continent. For example, a popular Web site in Europe may be slow to access for many North American users. Hence a mirror Web site may be set up in North America, which duplicates the content of the original site.

modem A device that allows your computer to communicate with another computer over a regular telephone line. Modems are often identified by the speed (in bits per second or bps) of communication they allow. The higher the bps, the faster the modem.

moderated Used in reference to either mailing lists or newsgroups. A moderated forum is one in which every message sent to that forum is first reviewed by an individual, often referred to as the "moderator." If the message is appropriate to the forum's topic, it is then approved and published on that forum. If it is not accepted for publication, the author is notified and the message is returned to the author. *See also* **open** and **closed**.

MPEG, Motion Picture Experts Group A standard for compressing digital video images.

NetPhone Also known as "Internet telephone." Refers to the software used to allow two individuals to talk to one another using the Internet as the connection.

Netiquette Rules of etiquette for online interactions. *See* `http://www.albion.com/netiquette/` for more detailed information.

newsgroups Also known collectively as "Usenet." Public discussion groups where individuals can read and add new messages (or "articles"). Uses a hierarchical topic structure (or "threads") to ease navigation through them. Messages posted to newsgroups are sent to every computer connected to the Internet, where the article is then stored for a few days to give people an opportunity to read it. Individual users elect to subscribe or not subscribe to newsgroups. While there are currently over 18,000 newsgroups available for subscription, most users only subscribe to, read, and contribute to a handful of them. A common way to carry on topic-specific discussion online; the other is via **mailing lists**.

newsgroup reader   The software used to access, read, and post to newsgroups.

open   In reference to a mailing list. An open mailing list allows anyone to post a message to it, regardless of whether they are a member of that list. *See also* **closed** and **moderated**.

operating system   The underlying system software that allows a computer to operate. Popular types of operating systems include DOS, Windows, and Macintosh System 7, 8, or X.

operator   A symbol or word used to help broaden or limit a search query. A specific type of operator, called a "Boolean operator," includes words such as `and`, `or`, and `not`.

PDF, Portable Document Format   Allows you to read a document and print it out using Adobe's Acrobat reader, a free piece of software. PDF files can *only* be read or printed using this software.

post   The act of adding a new message or article to a newsgroup, conference, or mailing list discussion area online.

PPP, Point to Point Protocol   A type of computer protocol used by modems for online communication.

protocol   A system of rules and procedures governing communications between two computer devices. File-transfer protocols in your communications program refer to a set of rules governing how error checking will be performed on blocks of data.

RAM, Random Access Memory   The temporary memory area on a computer that allows you to run software. Often increasing the amount of RAM in a computer can help poor computer performance.

RTF, Rich Text Format   A set of word processing instructions that can be read by most word processing programs, to retain the formatting rules of the document.

search engine   A Web site that indexes an online resource and makes that index available to others for searching. Most often in reference to a site that has indexed Web documents, but search engines also index mailing lists and other online resources. An "internal" search engine has only indexed the documents of that particular Web site, which can allow you to find information on that site more easily and quickly.

server   A computer dedicated to providing specific services to other computers. Print servers, for example, do nothing but accept, store, and print out documents sent to them by other computers. Web servers allow users from around the world to access the Web sites and documents stored on them.

shareware   Computer software that users are encouraged to copy and distribute to others, and to evaluate for a specified or indefinite period. The author gives the user a license to "try before you buy," and requires voluntary payment of a specific sum of money if the user continues to use the software. Failure to pay the requested fee is a legal violation of the author's copyright.

site   An area or location online, usually on the Web, where an organization, individual or business stores its information.

SLIP, Serial Line Internet Protocol   A type of computer protocol used by modems for online communication.

spam   Off-topic messages (usually advertisements) sent to a wide range of discussion forums (mailing lists or newsgroups) or e-mail addresses online. "Spamming" is frowned on in the online world.

T1   A kind of telephone line service offering high-speed data or voice access.

telnet   An application program that allows users to interactively logon to any computer on the Internet. For example, a telnet program could be used to search the holdings of a library and receive results.

thread   Messages on a single, specific topic that appear in the order they were written in an online discussion forum, such as on a newsgroup. Threads allow for easier reading of a particular subject, since they are all grouped together.

upload   Transfering files or software from your computer to another computer.

URL, Uniform Resource Locator   A format for an address on the Internet. For example, `http://www.cape.org/` indicates a Hypertext Transport Protocol (http) address on the World Wide Web (www) with location "cape" and the type of owner (org). Other valid protocols may include **ftp** and **gopher**. URLs are always sensitive to whether letters are in upper- or lowercase; that is, they are case sensitive.

user interface   The visual and design elements of a Web page that instruct users on how to access the Web site's information.

V.32bis   International standard for modem data communications at speeds of up to 14,400 bits per second.

V.34 International standard for modem data communications at speeds of up to 28,800 bits per second. Look for this designation when purchasing a new modem.

V.FC, V.Fast Class A pre-V.34 proprietary modem modulation for 28.8 Kbps connections, which is no longer a supported standard.

Web browser *See* **browser**.

Web log An online journal that is easily and regularly updated (usually daily or weekly), providing commentary and information through linking to other Internet resources, articles, and sites. It usually covers only a specific topic, such as technology, politics, or psychology. You may find Web log indexes at `http://www.blogger.com/`, `http://www.livejournal.com/`, and `http://www.moveabletype.org/`

Webmaster The person responsible for the ongoing maintenance of a Web site.

wildcard Most often an asterisk (*), a wildcard symbol allows you to tell the computer that you're uncertain what you're searching for. It can be used to ensure a search turns up all forms or variants of a word (e.g., `chil*` will turn up both `child` and `children`).

World Wide Web Also known as "the Web" or "WWW." A network of graphical hypertext servers linked by the Internet offering graphics, sound, text, and in some cases video clips providing information. This is the newest (since 1993) and fastest growing aspect of the Internet because of its ability to offer more than just plain text online.

XML, eXtensible markup language A higher-level language, similar to **HTML**, XML describes the content or data in a document, rather than how it is to be formatted. When companies in a single field, such as health care, all agree upon a single set of data definitions, they can then more easily exchange and find relevant information.

.zip An extension for a file name indicating the file is catalogued and compressed using Phil Katz's PKZIP compression utilities. You need a program called "pkunzip.exe" to decompress and extract the programs within this file.

APPENDIX B
Further Reading

Birnbaum, M. (2000). *Psychological Experiments on the Internet*. New York: Academic Press.

Calishain, T., & Dornfest, R. (2003). *Google Hacks: 100 Industrial-Strength Tips & Tools*. Cambridge, MA: O'Reilly & Associates.

Ewing, K., Reinhold, A., Levin Young, M., & Levine, J. (Eds.). (2002). *Internet All in One Desk Reference for Dummies* (2nd ed.). New York: Hungry Minds, Inc.

Ferguson, T. (1996). *Health Online*. Reading, MA: Addison-Wesley.

Gackenbach, J. (1998). *Psychology and the Internet: Intrapersonal, Interpersonal, and Transpersonal Implications*. New York: Academic Press.

Goss, S., & Anthony, K. (2003). *Technology in Counselling and Psychotherapy: A Practitioner's Guide*. Hampshire, UK: Palgrave Macmillan.

Kent, P. (2001). *The Complete Idiot's Guide to the Internet* (4th ed). Indianapolis, IN: Alpha Books.

Krug, S. (2000). *Don't Make Me Think! A Common Sense Approach to Web Usability*. Indianapolis, IN: Que Corporation.

McFedries, P. (2002). *Complete Idiot's Guide to Creating a Web Page* (5th ed.). Indianapolis, IN: Alpha Books.

McGuire, M., Stilborne, L., McAdams, M., & Hyatt, L. (2002). *The Internet Handbook for Writers, Researchers, and Journalists*. New York: Guilford Press.

Schlein, A., Sankey, M., & Newby, J. J. (Eds.). (2002). *Find It Online: The Complete Guide to Online Research* (3rd ed.). New York: Facts on Demand Press.

Wallace, P. (2001). *The Psychology of the Internet*. Cambridge, MA: Cambridge University Press.

White, B.J., Madara, E.J. (Eds.). (2002). *The Self-Help Sourcebook: Your Guide to Community & Online Support Groups* (7th ed.). Denville, NJ: Northwest Covenant Medical Center.

APPENDIX C
How to Get Online

Getting online—if you aren't already—is an easier task than you might imagine. You will need three things: a computer, a modem, and some type of online service provider.

THE COMPUTER

Virtually any computer can be turned into a connected online computer. You probably already have a computer or are thinking of getting one soon. Nearly any computer manufactured or purchased within the past 5 years will suffice. It can be something as old as an Intel-based Pentium or Pentium II machine (even older machines work, but at much slower speeds). Always try to purchase the highest megaherz (Mhz) machine you can afford, with the largest amount of storage space (40 gigabyte hard drives are not uncommon in new machines nowadays, something unheard of only 3 years ago). You should also look to purchase the largest amount of memory you can afford in your new machine, with a minimum of 64 megabytes (MB), but 128 MB of memory is even better for today's resource-intensive applications.

Do not worry if you cannot afford the fastest machine or processor available today, or the differences between an Intel Pentium III, IV, or Celeron, or AMD Athlon, or Duron chips. You will undoubtedly pay a large premium for the fastest processor available and will notice little difference in your ability to surf the Internet or run other common applications. For most people, the difference between a 600 Mhz Pentium chip and a 1.0 Ghz Pentium chip is difficult to gauge. Purchasing a cheaper, slower computer now will not make a significant difference down the road, as fewer people are upgrading their computers and operating systems every time a new operating system version is released from Microsoft. Few innovations have made their way to the average home user in the area of personal computer for the past 6 years, and this is unlikely to change any time soon.

Upgrading your existing computer is only an option if you are comfortable in messing with the internals of your computer or use a knowledgeable computer consultant. Computer upgrades, when all is taken into account, often are no more economical than purchasing a brand new, low-end (but usually more powerful) computer.

An Apple Macintosh computer is another, usually more expensive, option to consider. Macs' reputation for user-friendliness and being impossible to break in daily computing tasks has largely been surpassed within the PC world. The newest Macs *do* break (or "crash," in computer parlance), and the latest version of the Microsoft Windows operating system easily matches the capabilities found within Mac's OS X. In deciding between these two families, it is a decision largely based upon emotions than facts. Fewer software applications exist for the Mac, and hardware is available only from Apple itself (which means you will be dependent on them to set reasonable prices for such hardware). Test driving the two platforms can help you make a decision between them.

Minimum Computer Requirements

You should have at least a Pentium-class computer running at 133 Mhz to surf online. Memory is also an important factor, but it is somewhat dependent on your operating system. For older Windows-based machines, 32 megabytes (Mb) is usually sufficient; for Windows 95/98/ME, 64 megabytes is the minimum, and Windows NT/2000/XP operates best at 128 megabytes or more. A Macintosh II, Quadra, Performa, PowerPC, G3, G4, or iMac of any kind will work best in the Apple Macintosh world, with at least 32 Mb of RAM for Macintosh System 8, 9, or X (although 64 Mb is recommended). On any computer you use, you generally should have about 100 Mb of hard drive space available or free.

THE MODEM

A modem allows your computer to communicate with another computer over a regular telephone line. Most computers nowadays come with modems, but you can easily add one if necessary. Modem speed is usually the slowest link between you and the online world, so keeping up with the faster speeds within a year or two after they come out is usually a good idea. Modem speeds are measured in bits per second (bps); higher bps means a faster modem. You should get the fastest modem speed available at the time you buy. The newest, fastest modems are usually expensive in the first few months they're available, and then the price drops drastically. A minimum of a 28.8 Kbps modem is recommended for using the Internet, although 56 Kbps modems are standard and recommended.

If you're planning to spend a lot of time online or do daily business through an online connection, there is another option besides using your modem over a regular telephone line—a broadband connection. Broadband refers to a set of technologies that provide high-speed access to your home or office. It comes in a number of flavors—such as a cable modem, digital subscriber line (DSL), or ISDN—depending on which service is available to your location. It is commonplace that only one of these services will be available to your home or office. All three options offer high-speed access to the Internet, although cable modems and DSL are the least expensive (usually around $50/month, which includes the Internet service provider fee you would usually pay). Cable modems operate on your existing cable connection, whereas DSL connections operate on your existing telephone line. ISDN requires installation of a separate telephone connection, but may be the only technology available to some.

THE ONLINE SERVICE PROVIDER

There are dozens of ways to get online and access any of the resources discussed within this book. These include big commercial services, national or local Internet Service Providers (ISPs), your company or academic institution, or a "free-net."

Commercial Services

A common and popular method is to use one of the big commercial services, such as America OnLine (AOL) or CompuServe. The benefits to using one of these services include easy software installation and setup of your computer and modem. You not only will get good customer service around the clock, but also additional online areas and content you could not access through the Internet alone. These areas often include content (*Oprah*, for instance, is on America OnLine, as is *Car & Driver* magazine), discussion areas, interactive real-time chat with other members (all services), and interactive real-time game playing. The user interface tends to be well designed in these services, where "ease of use" is the underlying concept. You also get access to the Internet, although this access may not be as complete as that from an Internet Service Provider.

Naturally, all of this additional content, customer service, and ease of use comes at a price. In the past, the price of commercial providers has traditionally been higher than that of other commercial service providers offering only access to the Internet. But that has changed as more people have gotten online. Now these commercial services offer pricing that is usually competitive with Internet Service Providers (ISPs, see below). The other big drawback to using one of the commercial services is that their Internet access tends to be slower than if you were to access the Internet directly. This is due to the fact that you are accessing the Internet through the same computers as the commercial service's other 10 or 15 million subscribers. The providers try to reduce this traffic problem by using some software tricks (such as making copies of the most popular Web pages and serving them directly off of their machines instead of allowing the user to access the Web page directly), but it often isn't enough. The other common complaint I hear about accessing the Internet through these services is the number of times they *can't* be accessed due to busy signals. No matter how great an online service provider is, if you can't reach the online world through them, you won't remain a customer of them for long.

Internet Service Providers

Alternatives to the big three services come in the form of Internet Service Providers (ISP). ISPs may be nationally recognized companies providing Internet access or they may be a local company providing the same access. Typically this access includes not only the usual e-mail address and access to the Web and Internet newsgroups, but also the ability to set up your own Web page without any additional charge. Average charges for most areas of the country for these services range from $9.95 to $24.95 per month (at this writing), for unlimited access time while online. There usually is little difference in terms of the quality of services offered, busy signals, and other similar measurements between a national and a local ISP. However, national ISPs may not have a local phone number in your city or geographical location. You may have to select a local ISP to save on any long distance charges. Local ISPs can give more personalized service, but if something goes wrong on Saturday, they may not get around to fixing the problem until Monday; national ISPs often offer 24-hour customer service.

The other advantage to national over local Internet Service Providers is that—like commercial services—they will often provide you with all the necessary software to get started. This often comes on a CD-ROM that you simply load into your computer and follow their instructions. Compare this with many local ISPs. You may be given a diskette with a number of different programs on it and minimal, photocopied instructions (or worse yet, a "`readme.txt`" file on the diskette itself!). If you are knowledgable and comfortable with configuring your computer to use the programs, this software is usually enough to get you started; but because this can sometimes be a bit complicated, it is not recommended for the computer novice.

Workplace and Institutional Access

A third common way for people to access the online world is through their workplace or academic institution. However, unless it is a part of their job, I would caution clinicians accessing online resources from their workplace. Inappropriate or overuse of online surfing at work has been the cause of many supervisory meetings with employees. Check with your employer to see if they have a policy in place about online use. Universities and colleges have traditionally offered unlimited online access to faculty, staff, and students at no cost, not only from their offices and dorm rooms, but also from your home. With either of these means of access, you'll be able to get to all of the traditional online resources, including the Web, e-mail, and Internet newsgroups. What you may not get is any type of customer service or help in answering your technical questions. Online access speed may also be slower at some universities, because their connection to the Internet can't adequately support the number of simultaneous users at the institution. This is especially true when all of the students decide to go online at the same time!

Free-nets

Free-nets are the last typical method for accessing online resources. A free-net is exactly what it sounds like—a free way of accessing the Web, e-mail, and newsgroups. Often sponsored by local governments and administered through the public library, they grant an account to anybody who asks for one. Terminals are usually available on a first-come, first-served basis. Many of these types of services offer only rudimentary access, for instance, e-mail, newsgroups, and gopher access. As their budgets increase, many offer expanded services that rival a local ISP's, including Web access and your own Web page.

Which Provider Is Best for You?

I encourage people to start out with the easiest method for getting online—a commercial service—and see how they like it. Many times, staying with such a service is appropriate. For people who just want to access e-mail and the occasional Web site, such a commercial service is probably adequate. For others who do more serious Web surfing and make use of online Web technologies (such as Java, RealAudio, Web chat systems and the like), a direct Internet connection through an Internet Service Provider is a better long-term choice. Academic and work accounts are fine (and usually free), but you will often lose access to such accounts when you leave the university or employer. This loss of service may also come with little warning and with no guarantee of giving you time to transfer or copy personal files or e-mail you may have been saving. It's always a good idea to learn of your institution's policy on such matters before the time comes. In the meantime, enjoy the free account and make use of the unlimited access that comes with it. Whatever method you choose, don't become emotionally attached to it. Since the online world changes so quickly—and sometimes, drastically—be prepared to go with a better deal if one comes around.

APPENDIX D
Creating Your Own Web Resource

Creating your own World Wide Web site may seem like an enormous, expensive, and difficult undertaking. In fact, your own Web site can be online and functioning in less than a half hour once you master the basics of Web creation. Those basics are not as complicated as you may think.

Many programs exist to help you create your own Web presence. You can then choose to publish your Web page (or pages) on your Internet Service Provider's machine, or through one of the handful of free sites online, such as Yahoo!'s GeoCities (`http://geocities.yahoo.com/home/`). Once your site is online and you can access it through the Web, so can the millions of other individuals throughout the world connected to the Internet.

People choose to set up Web sites for a multitude of reasons. Clinicians often like to publish an advertisement for their practice or place of business, detailing their philosophical orientation for psychotherapy treatment, insurance accepted, business hours, other services offered, etc. Academicians or researchers may want to share their research interests with others, using their Web site as a publishing platform for their articles and theories. Other professionals simply would like a place to publish links to some of their favorite places online, or start a site that will act as a clearinghouse for online information in their particular specialty area in mental health.

There are two common ways to create a Web site. The simplest method is to choose what is called a "visual editor." The second method is to edit the language behind a Web page manually. Choosing the latter method means learning Hypertext Markup Language (HTML). HTML is *not* a programming language, such as BASIC or perl. Instead, it is similar to the insertion of formatting codes, such as that seen when a person chooses to "Reveal Codes" in the popular WordPerfect word processor. It specifies only how to display text in a Web browser. You tell it that a headline is a headline and it enlarges the font used, centers, and bolds the text on a person's Web browser. You tell it a paragraph ends here, and it places a blank line between two paragraphs. It is really that simple, regardless of whether you learn HTML or use the simpler visual editor.

There are dozens of software applications available on the market today to help you author Web pages in HTML. Some of these are free to download from select Web sites and many others are shareware, where you pay a fee only if you continue to use the program. This is certainly one of the easiest methods to use for creating a new Web page. Some popular word processors also allow you to publish a word processing document as an HTML document. My experience with leaving it to the word processor to make the translation has suggested that this is a good start to publishing a Web site. But you may need to go back and manually edit the HTML document anyway, because of problems in the translation. To supplement this wealth of programs available, I would also suggest buying a good book on the subject. See the bibliography for some of my suggestions.

Among the most popular Web building software, Microsoft's FrontPage (`http://www.microsoft.com/frontpage/`) and Macromedia's Dreamweaver (`http://www.macromedia.com/software/dreamweaver/`) are two of the easiest to use. Allaire's HomeSite product (`http://www.macromedia.com/software/homesite/`) is also worth your consideration. These programs make short work of building a professional and attractive Web site, in as little as a few hours. Most of this kind of software works just like a word processor—you just position images and text on a page, showing you what the finished page looks like as you create it. You don't even need to use a specialized editor such as these; any text editor (such as Notepad in Windows) will work just as well. That's because HTML is nothing but plain text. For instance, this is a Web page that will print the words, "Hello World!":

```
<html>
<head>
    <title>Type in your document title here</title>
```

```
</head>
<body>
        <div align="center">
                <h1>Hello world!</h1>
                <a href="http://grohol.com/">This is a
                link to my homepage</a>
        </div>
</body>
</html>
```

You'll notice that each HTML code (also referred to as HTML "tags") has a start and an end. Look at the "title" tag, for example. The ending tag for a particular HTML tag always begins with a regular slash (/). Not all HTML tags require an end tag, but most do. The specifics of what each tag means and what it does is more detailed than what I can go into here. I suggest either going to a good online reference for further explanation (see Yahoo! below) or purchasing a beginner's guide to HTML authoring (see the bibliography). Save your file with a "HTM" (Windows) or "HTML" (Macintosh) extension (e.g., "myfile.htm" or "myfile.html").

A Web page typically is made up of graphics and links to other Web sites as well. You can obtain graphics, as well as a great deal of additional authoring tips and tutorials, from dozens of online resources that have been developed to help new Web authors. Check a general subject guide, such as Yahoo! (http://www.yahoo.com/) for the links to these resources. You may link to any page online today *without* asking that page's owner for permission to do so. This allows you to create a Web page full of useful links to you on nearly any topic you'd like. It is also what makes the World Wide Web much like the spider's web, in that every Web page is linked to dozens or hundreds of others.

The most common question I receive after someone authors a Web page is, "What do I do with it now?" Well, one of the things you can do with it is open it up in your Web browser to see how it looks (if you haven't done so already). You can do this in Windows-based browsers by choosing the "File" menu, then the "Open File . . ." option. Specify the location of the HTML file and the name of it, and it will appear in your browser.

But how do you put it somewhere where others can access it? In order to do this, you will need to upload the file to a *Web server*. A Web server is a computer that serves Web pages. GeoCities (mentioned above) makes this easy for you, in that you just go to a specific place on their Web site and they walk you through this process, step by step. Others servers and Internet Service Providers have different procedures which vary. One common method is to use a piece of software called "ftp." ftp allows you to transfer a file between your computer and the Web server. You can get ftp through Shareware.Com (`http://www.shareware.com/`), which has further instructions on how to use it.

Index of Web Sites

Page numbers followed by "f" indicate figures; those followed by "t" indicate tables.

General Index

Page numbers followed by "f" indicate figures; those followed by "t" indicate tables.

315